Sweeping the Dust

For Glendy,
wishing you all
the best,
Lady Ruth

Lantern Books has elected to print this title on Rolland Enviro, a 100% post-consumer recycled paper, processed chlorine-free. As a result, we have saved the following resources:

12 trees, 332 lbs of solid waste, 31,31,427 gallons of water, 47 million BTUs of energy, 730 lbs of net greenhouse gases.

As part of Lantern Books' commitment to the environment we have joined the Green Press Initiative, a non-profit organization supporting publishers in using fiber that is not sourced from ancient or endangered forests. We hope that you, the reader, will support Lantern and the GPI in our endeavor to preserve the ancient forests and the natural systems on which all life depends. One way is to buy books that cost a little more but make a positive commitment to the environment not only in their words, but in the paper that they are published on. For more information, visit www.greenpressinitiative.org.

green press INITIATIVE

Sweeping the Dust

Ruth Lauer-Manenti

Lantern Books • New York
A Division of Booklight Inc.

2010
Lantern Books
128 Second Place
Brooklyn, NY 11231
www.lanternbooks.com

Printed in the United States of America

Library of Congress Cataloging-in-Publication Data

Lauer Manenti, Ruth.
Sweeping the dust / Ruth Lauer-Manenti.
p. cm.
ISBN-13: 978-1-59056-231-4 (alk. paper)
ISBN-10: 1-59056-231-3 (alk. paper)
1. Yoga. I. Title.
BL1238.52.L38 2010
294.5'436--dc22

2010029725

I bow down to the lotus feet of my guru Sri K. Pattabhi Jois

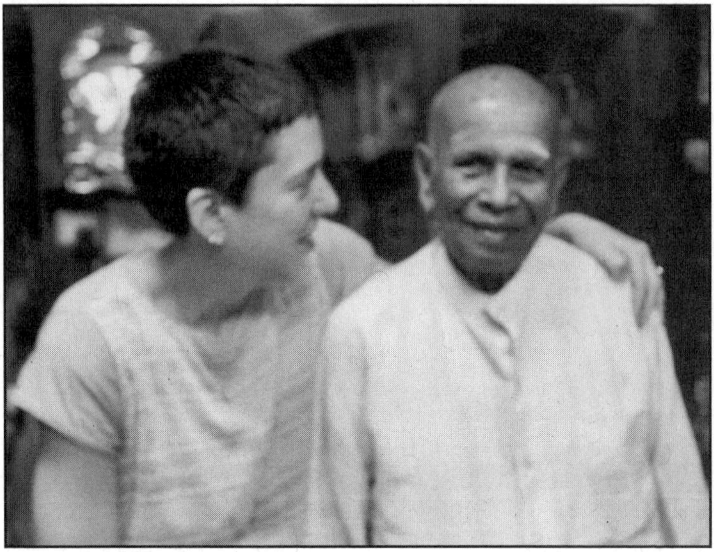

I dedicate this book to my guru Sri K. Pattabhi Jois,
his daughter Saraswathi Jois and grandson Sharath Jois,
to my teachers Sharon Gannon and David Life,
to my teachers Dr. M. A. Jayashree, and Prof. M. A. Narasimhan,
to my parents Stefanie and Lothar Lauer,
and to my husband Robert Manenti.

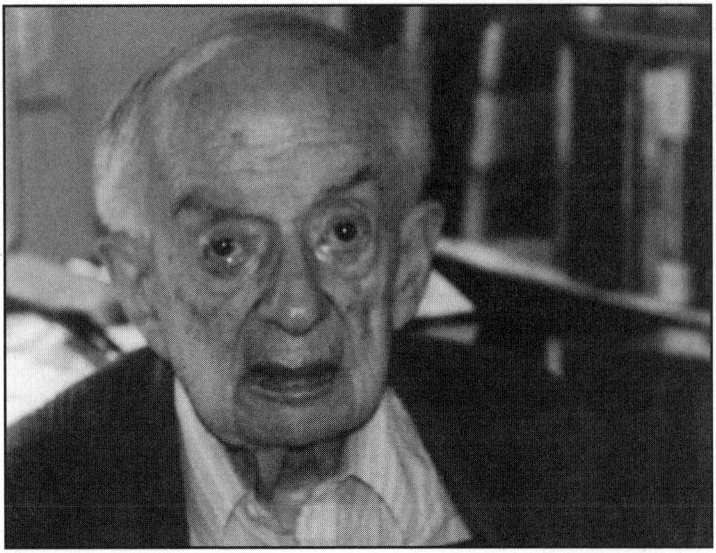

For my father. I miss you.

For Andrea. I swept because she brought the broom.

Acknowledgments

This book is a collection of teachings inspired by monthly essays written by my teacher Sharon Gannon, and that were given at the Jivamukti Yoga School in New York City to a group of students who have stuck by me for some time now. Their presence in my life demands that I grow as a teacher, which ensures that I won't spend too much time in my robe and slippers, watching TV. I am most grateful to this group. Students usually think that it is they who love the teacher, but actually it is mutual.

Of course, without the Jivamukti Yoga School there would never have been what has been and is, on so many levels, wonderful. For that, I thank my teachers David Life and Sharon Gannon. They are saints, their words have power, their prayers come true, and their blessings are holy. Traditionally, one sought the blessing of the elder or the wise one. I feel their blessing in my life all the time. They gave me their blessing for this book.

I want to thank my student Rima Rabbath for following me with a tape recorder, an iPod, a Blackberry, and now a microchip. Her belief that what I would say would be worth recording made it worth recording.

I want to thank my student Andrea Boyd. It is difficult for me to express my gratitude to someone who has worked so hard on my behalf. Sometimes, I really think she did all the work; but, actually, we collaborated. We shared.

I want to thank Jessica Kung, Stéphane Dreyfus, Charlotte Hamilton, Reema Datta, and Eve Smith for their input on, and laying out of, the Sanskrit, so we could have the verses in the original alphabet. Even if one can't read Sanskrit, the language is visually beautiful. I feel honored to have such beauty in my book.

I want to thank Jordan Tinker for scanning the artwork that appears on the cover as well as the inside photos. The high quality gives the book an especially pleasing appearance.

I want to thank my mother, Stefanie Lauer, for doing the final editing. Having her hand in the book gave me piece of mind.

I want to thank my publisher, Martin Rowe. His support gives me a place to put my stories that might otherwise get lost. Again, I find myself in a position where it's difficult to express my gratitude.

Additional thanks to: Fern Manenti, Michael Lauer, Lisa Schrempp, Professor H. V. Nagaraja Rao, Dr. C. A. Gurudat, Ambika Gurudat, Geshe Michael Roach, Lama Christie McNally, Eddie Stern, Jeffrey Cohen, Ananda Ashram, The Pfister-Tinker Family, Kimberly Flynn, Lois Conner, Kelly Britton, Jessica Perry, Valerie Schaff, Jill Seslowsky, Monica Jaggi, Pamela Boyd, Carin DeNat, Manizeh Rimer, John and Connie Conroy, and Carlos Menjivar.

Contents

Acknowledgments *xiii*
Explanation of the Ancient Scriptures Used *xvii*
A Note about the Sanskrit *xx*
Foreword by Sharon Gannon *xxiii*
Introduction *xxvii*

Here and Now *1*
The Dalai Lama's Room *3*
A Very Old Harmonium *5*
Grow Wild *9*
I Turned on the TV *11*
Barley Balls *14*
O Happy Day *17*
Time Passed *20*
A Sweet Memory of Jayashree *23*
Contrasts and Metaphors *26*
Satkara *28*
The Airline Magazine *31*
Isis and the Yogi Take Forms *34*
Trust *36*
Holy Presence *39*
The Fabulous Mr. Roth *42*
Manhattan Skyline *44*

Saucha 47
Nothing Belongs to Us 49
For Asako 52
Sweeping the Dust 54
The Guru's Feet 56
Rainbow Falafel 58
Yoga Communities 62
Getting Yelled At 65
The Man with the Shaved Head in the Vegetable Section 68
Teacher's Training 71
Not Eating Meat 74
En Theos 76
A Blade of Grass 79
Precious Books 81
A Quality of Readiness 83
The Guru's Breath Count 86
The Jackfruit Tree 88
Brush with Death 91
Voices in Our Head 93
Refraining from Speaking 96
The Antidote to Unhappiness 99
For Steven 101
Life's Interruptions 103
One by One 105
My Father's Light 107
Going Forward in a Boat 109

About the Author 112

Explanation of the Ancient Scriptures Used

The Yoga Sutras

No one really knows when Master Patanjali compiled *The Yoga Sutra,* but the general consensus is sometime between 400 BCE to 400CE. Master Patanjali did not actually write *The Yoga Sutra,* rather he selected the essential teachings on yoga from the Vedas, some of the oldest books in the world. He stitched them together and called it *The Yoga Sutra.* Sutra means thread or stitch. Each sutra relates to the ones that come before and after it, one continuous thread, therefore it is called *The Yoga Sutra,* and not *The Yoga Sutras.* There are four chapters and 195 sutras, in which we find the crux of yoga philosophy and practice: how to uncover the light of awareness, obscured by the bias and irritation of the individual, so that one may stop superimposing conditioning on everything and see the underlying sameness of all beings. The sutras are concise, as it was expected that they would be memorized. Each one is said to be "packed," implying that a teacher would be needed to help in the "unpacking." The difficulty in digging out the meaning of the sutras trains the mind to dig into oneself and find what is there.

There are various accounts about Master Patanjali's birth. One is that he fell (*pat*) from the heavens into the palms (*anjali*) of a childless woman who was praying to become pregnant. He fell in the form of a snake with a thousand heads (*Adishesha*), each head representing a *pandit* (spiritual teacher). It is said that at the time of his birth he caused his mother no pain. Such is also the case in the birth stories of the Buddha and Jesus.

The Bhagavad Gita

A long time ago, perhaps 2100 BCE, there was a warrior named Arjuna who was destined to go to war with his family, and was despondent. For guidance he went to the lord, Sri Krishna, who was said to be a full incarnation of Vishnu, the god of preservation. The dialogue takes place on a battlefield, which is synonymous with the challenges we face during life and the fight that goes on within one's mind.

Found in the *Bhishma Parva,* the middle section of the *Mahabharata, The Bhagavad Gita,* or "The Song of the Lord" has eighteen chapters. Around the fourth century BCE, Vyasa, the great Vedic poet, used his divine powers to put the story into 700 verses, sometimes called the "700 suns" that dispel the darkness of ignorance. Written in conversational style, the verses are set to meter, and can be sung in temples, caves, villages, and cities, as a form of study, prayer, while working, before eating, waiting for the bus, or anytime. The beauty of the poetry is often compared to the petals of the lotus flower in bloom.

In the verses, the teacher gives the student a way of living that removes suffering—emphasizing kindness, equanimity, karma, renunciation, meditation, and duty. The student is taught to embrace the entire universe, to be easily approachable by others, and to be at home everywhere. The student of yoga is described as a devotee. Thus, the guidelines on the path (how to eat, sleep, work, and treat others) are not followed in a wearisome way, but with dedication and love.

When Arjuna's doubts are cleared, his neurosis ends, and ultimately he realizes Sri Krishna's knowledge as his own. Just as the parent wishes for the child to go further in life than he or she, or as the cow wishes for her calf a life free of suffering, the teacher wishes to be surpassed by their student. Thus Sri Krishna was fulfilled by Arjuna.

This book is known to be the one book that Mahatma Gandhi kept on his night table.

The Hatha Yoga Pradipika by Yogi Swatmarama was written between the sixth and fifteenth centuries CE. It is for the young or old, educated or uneducated. It defines yoga as a state of mind, where one's individual thoughts have been put aside and the mind is no longer caught in its own pursuits. This is referred to as a mindless or cosmic state of mind, *manomani*. This does not mean that a person becomes thoughtless. On the contrary, one actually sets an example by one's thoughtfulness, as one's mind is freed from thinking only of oneself. By a combined effort of putting the body in different postures (*asanas*), for example, standing on one's head; by holding one's breath or vital air for long periods of time (*pranayama*); by cleaning oneself from the inside (*kriya*), for example, pouring water in one nostril, tilting the head, and letting the water drip out the other nostril; by focusing the eyes at a single point like a candle flame so as to develop concentration (*tratak*); by leading an ethical life (*yama*) occupied in nonviolence (*ahimsa*), with a support system (*niyama*) of enthusiasm, perseverance, a positive attitude, and study of scripture—currents of energy move upwards and the yogi gets this mindless state of mind.

Through these practices (*abhyasa*), and the grace of a guru, or teacher, one is able to drive away the impurities and purify the subtle channels (*nadis*), which are pathways that energy (*shakti*) moves through. As the spinal pathway becomes clear, the yogi hears holy sounds (*nadam*). These sounds awaken previously dormant areas of the brain so that the yogi stops seeing one as two, there are no distinctions between subject and object, and one exists not as a separate individual but as part of a whole, in a reality that is indivisible. Herein we find the basis of Vedanta philosophy, and hundreds of thousands of sentences in hundreds of thousands of books on the unity in all things. Duality and otherness, us and them, dissolve like salt into water.

The rising of this snakelike energy (*kundalini*) from the base of the spine and ending slightly above one's head transforms the yogi. Negative traits or tendencies within his or her personality disappear permanently and he or she is likened to a lotus flower with one thousand petals. Eventually, the energy moves with such speed that a pin-size hole is pierced at the top of the head and God drips down through it in the form of nectar (*amrit*), thus opening the yogi's third eye at the ajna chakra, the point between the eyebrows. One sees the interconnectedness of life, and in that sees God. Absorbed in a greater consciousness, the yogi and anyone in his vicinity are happy. By following the instructions of the guru well and keeping a vegetarian diet, the practitioner frees him- or herself from fatigue, wipes out diseases, and ultimately skips death.

A Note about the Sanskrit

Most of the teachings that follow begin with a Sanskrit verse—the spoken knowledge of sages, written down in books and preserved as scriptures. The translations are not word-for-word. Rather, they are poetic interpretations I arrived at through the grace and influence of the following masters: Shri Brahmananda Saraswati, I. K. Taimni, Sri Swami Satchidananda, S. Radhakrishnan, Swami Muktibodhananda, Winthrop Sargeant, and Swami Prabhupada.

I found the following sources useful for the Sanskrit *devanagari* script and transliteration:

- *The Yoga Sutras of Patanjali* by Sri Swami Satchidananda
- *Bhagavad Gita, As It Is* by A. C. Bhaktivedanta Prabhupada
- *God Talks with Arjuna: The Bhagavad Gita,* by Paramahansa Yogananda
- *The Hatha Yoga Pradipika* by Dr. M. A. Jayashree
- *Sabda-Dhatumanjari* by Dr. M. A. Jayashree
- *Jivamukti Yoga School Chant Book* by Sharon Gannon
- Yoga Studies Institute Course Materials by Geshe Michael Roach and Lama Christie McNally

Foreword

Sharon Gannon

I would call Ruth Lauer-Manenti a very "hip" person, in the best sense of that term, because she is in the now. The word hip refers to something or someone who is current, who has something relevant to say to us now. Ruth is a living example of the type of person whom mystic poet William Blake described as one who can "see a world in a grain of sand / And a heaven in a wild flower." She looks deeply into the ordinary world and, in doing so, magically transforms the ordinary into the extraordinary. Or rather, she reveals to us that it was never mundane in the first place but was always a magical place of infinite possibilities, if we were only willing to look deeper.

Sweeping the Dust is a living testament to what Patanjali expresses in his opening of the Yoga Sutra: *atha yoganushasanam,* which can be translated as, "Now this is yoga as I have observed it in the natural world." This opening line is profound on many levels and can be seen as a riddle or a Zen koan, with the whole of yoga contained in the seed of that first sutra. Significantly, Patanjali says *atha,* which means "now"—not "once upon a time." This is very encouraging, because when anyone opens this holy scripture and reads that first sutra and that first word, automatically yoga has relevance to that person: it's about them; it has implications for the life they are living right at that moment. Atha brings it into the world of the living, rendering it current—hip—right now. *Yoganushasanam* means that yoga can be found all around us in the natural world, if we are willing to look deeper into things, and not if we are content to live on the surface. That is just what Ruth does with these seemingly simple little vignettes taken from her real life and everyday experiences.

Ruth shares with us the fruit of her yogic ability to *tanu*—to stretch her mind and draw deep insights from living an examined life. She looks into the world around her to find yoga. This relative world is composed of many *jivas* or individuated atomic beings. The word *anu* from *anushasanam* means atom—the minute, mostly indivisible parts that make up the whole. For a yogi—one who can step into the present moment of now—all atoms (separate component parts) can be seen as yoked together making up the whole. Every encounter has profound meaning, providing a means to link one to the infinite. This is what it means to see the world as a whole, or "holy" place. The methods of yoga refine our perception, allowing us to explore this possibility.

Ruth says that "Sweeping the Dust" is a metaphor—a way of saying that taking care of the ground has value. The ground of being, the natural world, forms the foundation for our lives. The material that we stand on and that surrounds us every day and that is often taken for granted—the seemingly small and insignificant aspects of life—are important if we know how to look and what to look for.

I often speculate on how Ruth's childhood must have been, growing up with a poet for a mother and a physicist for a father, as she most definitely is a combination of the two rich worlds of Art and Science. She delights in probing into the sub-atomic world of feeling to discover the relationships that might connect a simple touch on a shoulder to the celestial movements of the sun, moon, and stars. She juggles effortlessly with the lofty abstract and the unassuming mundane as if she were just calmly sweeping up the dust. She has a natural knack for stretching her mind and heart to include, rather than look for differences, and sees connections among things.

The stories in this book are all about seeing so deeply into things that you come out the other end. For instance, she writes about how eating a falafel can be *sadhana,* a spiritual practice, which can contribute to peace on earth; or if your heart aches when you hear about an earthquake in a faraway place it is called *bodhi chitta,* a Sanskrit word meaning "awakening"; or how being yelled at by someone who loves you has the power to dispel worry and anxiety; or how the beauty and poise of a dying cat, whose last action was to get up and use the litter box so as to not dirty her bed so that in the next moment she could lie down in a clean bed and die, teaches us about the importance of *saucha,* a yogic practice of keeping ourselves and our surroundings clean. Ruth shows us it is in the embracing of the little things, the natural everyday activities in which our soul has a chance to shine.

Once when I was in Mysore, India with Ruth we were walking down a dusty street and we passed the remains of a building that perhaps had been a hotel at one point in its past history. A second floor was still remaining but without walls or a roof, just a skeleton of old bamboo poles and a cement floor. However, there was a white, porcelain bathtub sitting there, amidst all the rubble. Ruth stopped and was enraptured, with eyes wide open, her head slowly nodding from side to side as she said something like, "so beautiful, look how it is just sitting there."

Ruth sees things differently than most of us, perhaps more magically, if by magic you mean when there is a shift in one's perception of the world. She is like a soul in wonder—every moment is filled with possibilities for going deeper into life, and because of that she is not only magical but also radical. The word radical, like the word radish, derives from the word *rad* meaning "root" (*rad* is also a slang word synonymous with hip or cool). A radical is someone who attempts to get at the root of a situation, to peel away all the superficial layers and uncover the core. Writer Joseph Conrad said, "One must explore deep and believe the incredible to find the new particles of truth floating in an ocean of insignificance." This is how Ruth lives her life. Fortunately she can also describe it in the most elegant and succinct ways, and that is what you, the reader, will discover when you read the pages of this book.

Introduction

पत्रं पुष्पं फलं तोयं यो मे भक्त्या प्रयच्छति ।
तदहं भक्त्युपहृतमश्नामि प्रयतात्मनः ॥ २६ ॥

patraṃ puṣpaṃ phalaṃ toyaṃ yo me bhaktyā prayacchati
tad ahaṃ bhakty-upahṛtam aśnāmi prayatātmanaḥ

Whatever is offered to me with a pure loving heart, no matter if it is as small as a leaf, a flower, a piece of fruit, or sip of water, I will accept it.

—THE BHAGAVAD GITA, CHAPTER NINE, VERSE 26

When I first went to India, I was eager to look at the Indian miniature paintings from the sixteenth century. I had seen many of them in museums in the West, and assumed that in India I would find the best collections. But the museums in India are poorly lit, so I couldn't see anything. What I did find, though, was incredible artistic beauty in a hand-painted spoon, the tapestry covering a chair, a clay cup, an embroidered shawl, a hand-woven man's skull cap, and carpets made from rags called rag-rugs. So I gave up looking for art in a museum and instead found it in daily life.

Worshiping is like this, also. We may look for God in the museum, church, or temple, but God is not limited to such places: He is everywhere. But how do we find God everywhere? By treating everyone as God. And how would God like to be treated? In this verse, the Lord says bring me a leaf, a flower, a fruit, or some water with devotion. He wants something unpretentious that expresses affection. If we can do this with everyone, we will know the meaning of this verse. One stick of incense, a single good word, food for one dog, memorizing one text, bowing down one time, or one warm cup of tea—all are acceptable to the Lord.

In 2009, my guru Sri K. Pattabhi Jois passed away. Shortly afterwards, I asked his daughter Saraswathi for something that had belonged to him. She presented me with an old and worn-out shawl. It was folded in her hands, and she extended it toward me saying, "It was Guruji's favorite. It is very simple. You will like it. He didn't like the fancy ones." This shawl, torn in several places, was a perfect offering. It greatly pleased me; in this way, Saraswathi had pleased the Lord. Pleasing the Lord releases us of tensions. Making me happy made her happy, even in the midst of such a sad time.

There is a man I know in India who doesn't have any legs; he is cut off from the hips down. He has a piece of wood he has tied himself to, and he pulls himself around with his arms. He sits in a spot I pass and asks for money, yelling, "Amma, Amma." He is calling me *mother*. He wants me to offer him kindness; he wants me to see God in those who suffer. Guruji once told me that that man was God, "disguised."

The word *asana* means a seat, something to lean on, a support. Offering someone support can take shape in a myriad of ways. These ways can be the threads that tie everything together. Offerings join the giver and the receiver spiritually.

Sadly, leaves, flowers, fruit, and water are disappearing as we destroy the earth. The best offering we can make in these times is to become vegetarian, a gentle diet that causes the least harm to plants, animals, the climate, and human beings. If we continue to clear away the forests, trees, shrubs, prairies, meadows, marshes, grasslands, plants, roots, flowers, creepers, and weeds, in order to grow one kind of crop to feed to animals who will be slaughtered, there won't be any more leaves, flowers, fruit, or water in our landscapes.

Scriptures are prophetic with obvious and not-so-obvious meanings. Perhaps the Lord is telling us in this verse that leaves, flowers, fruit, and water are offerings from the Lord for us to protect and offer back.

My husband Robert and I live in a cabin in the woods. Often, bees, wasps, flying ants, even an occasional snake come into our home. My husband knows how to handle these animals appropriately. Without upsetting them, he puts a container over them, slides a piece of paper underneath and carries them back outside.

Sweeping the Dust is a way of saying that taking care of the ground has value. Traditionally, the yogi has always sat on the ground. Only an elder or a greatly esteemed master would be given a chair. Everything rests on the ground. The ground is the support. It's where we can sit together and tell our stories. Sweeping the dust is a metaphor. In that spirit, I offer this book, like a tiny piece of Guruji's torn shawl.

Here and Now

अथ योगानुशासनम् ॥ १ ॥

atha yogānuśāsanam

Now this is Yoga observed in a tiny moment seated in the world.

—MASTER PATANJALI'S *YOGA SUTRAS*, BOOK ONE, SUTRA I

Atha means now. *Anushasanam* means within the world. Where is this yoga? It is within this world. When? Now.

A while ago, I received a phone call from my brother's sixteen-year-old son Nathan. Nathan had to write a paper for high school on *To the Lighthouse* by Virginia Woolf and said he didn't understand the book. He asked my brother for assistance, and my brother said, "You'll have to go to your aunt Ruth on that subject. It's one of her favorite books."

Nathan complained that there was no plot.

I said, "Let's not look for the plot. Let's feel for the essence of the story."

He said, "Okay. Well, what's the essence of the story?"

"It's not in the words, you see," I replied, "but the words are the clues to the essence of the story."

"Yeah? Like what?"

"For example, throughout the novel the main character in the book opens and shuts the windows," I continued. "It's like an aria, a chorus, an overture. She opens the windows, things happen, and then she shuts the windows. It's a main theme throughout."

"Yeah," he said.

"Did you notice that?"

"Maybe."

"When she opens the windows," I said, "it's to show she has a positive outlook about herself and others. She wants to invite the outer world in. When she shuts the windows, she feels fragile, vulnerable; she wants to hide and even feels some shame."

"Wow!" Nathan exclaimed. "Can you write my paper for me?"

"Nathan, don't worry. You'll do a great job," I said. "You just need to read more carefully."

"Okay," he said.

At the end of our conversation, I told him, "When you read, bow down to Virginia Woolf. Read in that mood: Have reverence for what you're reading."

Virginia Woolf is a great writer who can hone in on a detail to communicate something boundless. Through her artistry the specifics express a deeper meaning. The Lord does the same thing. Everything means more than its appearance. Everything is more than it seems. *Atha* is now, it's a small moment in time (*anu*) where one observes something vast in the world, like someone opening a window. Master Patanjali is saying, *Take notice, pay attention to your world.*

The Dalai Lama's Room

यज्ञदानतपःकर्म न त्याज्यं कार्यम् एव तत् ।
यज्ञो दानं तपश्चैव पावनानि मनीषिणाम् ॥ ५॥

yajñadānatapaḥkarma na tyājyaṃ kāryam eva tat
yajño dānaṃ tapaścaiva pāvanāni manīṣiṇām

The action involved in yajna, dana, and tapas verily ought to be performed, and should not be forsaken, for the holy fire rite, philanthropy, and self-discipline sanctify the wise.

—*THE BHAGAVAD GITA*, CHAPTER EIGHTEEN, VERSE 5

Tapas—to heat, to burn, to melt, to boil, hard work, austerities, self-discipline, to sweat, to persevere, to try again and again

In yoga *asana*, there is the principle of going down in order to rise up. We see this also in nature, where the bird presses down on the branch in order to fly. When a skyscraper is built, first the ground is dug into deeply, so that the foundation can support the height. It is a universal principle called "leverage." We surrender to something bigger than ourselves and it makes us light.

A few years back, there was a student in Mysore studying Ashtanga yoga with Sri K. Pattabhi Jois. This student was also studying Tibetan Buddhism in a town called Bylakuppe, two-and-a-half hours south of Mysore, where on account of the generosity of the Indian government a Tibetan community was established after the Tibetans had to flee their country. The Dalai Lama lives there when he is in southern India. This student arranged a trip for Guruji, who had never been to Bylakuppe, to see the monasteries and the murals inside them, to meet with the high lamas, and even to spend the night. A car came for Guruji.

When he returned from his visit, we were waiting for him in the foyer of his house.

"How was your trip to Bylakuppe?" we asked.

"Oh, Bylakuppe, I liking very much. Dalai Lama's people I liking. Good people. I staying Dalai Lama's room."

It turned out that the Dalai Lama hadn't been there, so the monks had decided to honor Guruji by inviting him to sleep in the Dalai Lama's own room. Guruji was very happy about this and said over and over again, "I staying Dalai Lama's room."

"What is the Dalai Lama's room like?" we asked.

"Oh, Dalai Lama's room, it is very good," Guruji said. "It is very simple. For sleeping, only one straw mat. Electricity not coming. Water not coming. Television not coming. Mosquitoes coming."

We think it's hard to live like that: not having every gadget, not having all the conveniences. But that's *tapas*—accepting some hardness as part of life as a blessing. You're not afraid to be uncomfortable. The Dalai Lama chooses to have the one straw mat. He's living simply and low to the ground. Simultaneously, His Holiness is leading a movement for world peace and uplifting himself and millions of others all around the world.

A Very Old Harmonium

देवान् भावयतानेन ते देवा भावयन्तु वः ।
परस्परं भावयन्तः श्रेयः परम् अवाप्स्यथ ॥ ११ ॥

devān bhāvayatānena te devā bhāvayantu vaḥ
parasparaṃ bhāvayantaḥ śreyaḥ param avāpsyatha

When humanity honors and cherishes the devas, the devas, in turn, will cherish and nourish humanity.

—*THE BHAGAVAD GITA*, CHAPTER THREE, VERSE 11

In 2009, I went to India. I had planned to study music and singing. I have a great teacher there named Dr. Gurudat. Dr. Gurudat has many students, from all different backgrounds and ages, who would come for their music lessons. If he is too busy with his other work of teaching law, his wife, Chandrika, gives the music lessons, and if she is busy, their daughter Ambika gives the lessons. Years ago, I had lessons with Ambika, who was only fourteen and already a master. The Gurudat family are all great musicians and gifted teachers. I consider myself extremely fortunate to study with them.

When I'm studying, the family loans me a harmonium to practice on. If I'm not practicing, I won't get far. But when I went to India in 2009, they didn't have a harmonium that I could use. Dr. Gurudat said, "I have a friend who has a little music shop in town, his name is Ramesh. I'll call him. Maybe he has a spare. He has a lot of instruments." Dr. Gurudat called Ramesh, who said I could come and pick up a harmonium. "Ramesh is expecting your call," said Dr. Gurudat. So I went to Ramesh's tiny shop and picked up the harmonium. It was in a bag and I thanked him and said that in a little more than a month I'd return it.

It turned out that the harmonium was very old. I could tell from looking at it. It was elegant and had a hauntingly beautiful sound. Never in my life had I played a harmonium that sounded so wonderful. I attributed this somewhat to its age. In the old days, they made things better. I loved having the harmonium and it motivated me to practice even more than I would have, because I loved its sound. At one point in the month I thought, "I'd like to own this." So I phoned and spoke with Ramesh's wife and said I really liked the harmonium and was wondering about maybe purchasing it. "That harmonium is not for sale," she said. The way she said it made me regret having asked. I thought I must have sounded crass.

When I was just about to leave India, I phoned Ramesh and said I would like to bring the harmonium back. He said, "Yes, come. Four o'clock." So I went to return the harmonium and Ramesh was there. "I don't sell the antique harmoniums," he said. "That harmonium you had was a hundred years old." Then he said, "I don't rent harmoniums. I don't rent them or loan them out. They're not for hire." He told me it was only because Dr. Gurudat had requested he give the harmonium to me that I had got it. He would do whatever Dr. Gurudat requested, and it was only for that reason that he had given me the harmonium. He kept repeating himself. "I don't rent. I don't rent. Not for sale. Very old. Very old. Hundred years old. Not for sale. Only for Dr. Gurudat. He is asking. He is asking."

Ramesh then went on to tell me how great Dr. Gurudat was, and what a high opinion he had of Dr. Gurudat. Of course, Dr. Gurudat had been my teacher for many years, so I knew how great Dr. Gurudat was. But, I love to be reminded. Ramesh was saying that Dr. Gurudat taught music to a lot of youths whose families couldn't afford musical lessons, and that he charged whatever they could give. The Gurudat family, Ramesh noted, lived simply, were great musicians, musical geniuses, gifted teachers, and a pure, kind, and traditional family. He couldn't express enough his regard for this family. It was only because of that, that he had given me the harmonium.

I wanted Ramesh to know that I agreed with him. I said, "Yes, the family is pure. They are perfect. I agree. I understand you made this exception for me. Thank you so much, I enjoyed having it." We came together, Ramesh and I, in that we both cherished Dr. Gurudat and loved and revered his family.

In this verse from *The Bhagavad Gita,* Sri Krishna, the Lord himself, is teaching his student Arjuna that the student shouldn't just cherish the music teacher, but that the student should cherish nature. Without nature we could not sustain ourselves, just like without the music teacher, I would not have had the harmonium.

Perhaps you are sitting on a floor made of bamboo. In order to grow, the bamboo needs the earth, the sun, and the rain, which makes it possible for us later to have a floor to sit on. The clothes that the yogi wears are cotton. Cotton grows in the earth, and the insects participate. Nature has a chain, and Sri Krishna is saying that you will reach a point in your *sadhana,* your yoga practice, that's deep enough for you to realize that everything is provided for you, and you will cherish that. In that realization, nature will be able to provide for you. She provides for the ones who cherish her. If we don't cherish nature, she cannot provide properly for us.

It is crucial that we honor her, acknowledge where everything comes from, and not be in denial. If we are thirsty, there is water. When we acknowledge where everything comes from, we become humble. When we sit at the table to eat our meal of vegetables provided for us, humility is there. It's through that humility and not through arrogance that we come to know ourselves and feel nourished. If we don't think about where things come from, we think, "Well, *I've* got that harmonium! It has nothing to do with Dr. Gurudat." So we have to be humble. That's our great fortune, to be humble.

Grow Wild

यावत् संजायते किंचित् सत्त्वं स्थावरजङ्गमम् ।
क्षेत्रक्षेत्रज्ञसंयोगात् तद् विद्धि भरतर्षभ ॥ २६ ॥

yāvat saṃjāyate kiṃcit sattvaṃ sthāvarajaṅgamam
kṣetrakṣetrajñasaṃyogāt tad viddhi bharatarṣabha

Whatever exists—every being, every object; the animate, the inanimate—understand that to be born from the union of nature and spirit.

—*THE BHAGAVAD GITA*, CHAPTER THIRTEEN, VERSE 26

A while ago, one of my students who is a fashion designer had a dream in which she gave a dress to Sharon Gannon, one of her yoga teachers. When my student awoke, she remembered the dress and created a whole line based on the one she had dreamed of. They were the most beautiful dresses in the world. Time passed, and I needed a dress for the party in honor of my first book, *An Offering of Leaves.* She asked me if I would accept one of her dresses. "You would be helping me to realize my dream," she said. The dress she gave me was sheer and multi-layered. It was ivory-colored and moved when I did, as if it were a part of me. The night I wore it, I felt like an angel with wings.

A week later, I was walking down the street in New York City when I came upon an elderly man who was trying to tie his shoelaces. He was standing on a busy street looking overwhelmed.

I wanted to help him. I used to tie my father's shoelaces all the time; it took great skill because his feet were always swollen. If I tied the laces too tight, he complained that I was cutting off his circulation; if I tied the laces too loosely, he complained that they could come undone and he might trip. Half the time he didn't want even to step outside, because he didn't want to put his shoes on. I became good at tying his shoes just right. It was something I loved to do, something that I can do no longer since my dad has passed away.

When I saw the old man on the street, I knew I could do a good job. I asked him if he needed help. "Yes," he replied. I found a ledge he could sit on, and then I squatted low on the ground. I liked being on the level of his shoes, where I could look up at him. I tied them really nicely, and he was happy and so was I. I felt as if I was tying my dad's shoes, even though it wasn't my dad. I thanked the elderly man, for he had helped me to be in touch with my father.

If I want to honor my father, I can walk around the world and tie the shoelaces of elderly people. But looking only for elderly people might mean overlooking the needs of others. We can help anyone at any time. This is what it means to be wild or natural. When things grow wild, they grow everywhere. A tree growing on one side of the fence may drop its fruit on the other side. The tree is not concerned with those kinds of boundaries.

It's natural to see my father everywhere. That is the wild side of my spirit—it knows no boundaries.

I Turned on the TV

इडा भगवती गङ्गा पिङ्गला यमुना नदी ।
इडा पिङ्गलयोर्मध्ये बाल रण्डा च कुण्डली ॥ ११० ॥

iḍā bhagavatī gaṅgā piṅgalā yamunā nadī
iḍā piṅgalayor madhye bāla raṇḍā ca kuṇḍalī

Within the human body there are thousands of energetic channels. Two major channels are the ida and the pingala. Ida is on the left side, called the Ganges, like the river. Pingala is on the right side, called the Yamuna, like the river. In the middle of the Ida and the Pingala is the infant widow, Kundali."

—THE HATHA YOGA PRADIPIKA,
CHAPTER THREE, VERSE 110

Some time ago, my spirits were low, and sometimes when my spirits are low, I look to see if there's anything worth watching on television. So I turned on the TV and went through my three channels and the Oprah Winfrey Show was on. I like Oprah very much so I decided to watch the program.

Oprah had a middle-aged woman as her guest, a very attractive and quite glamorous and fit-looking person. This woman had great posture, she was bubbly and glowing, her hair was shining, and she looked lovely. I was wondering who she might be. She had written a book called something like *21 Days to the Perfect Body and Perfect Health,* and she was on the show to tell Oprah about it.

Then came the commercial break. I expected the show to be good and believed that I'd enjoy watching it.

When the show came back on, the guest explained the diet: no meat, no dairy, no animal products, no sugar (that would be hard for me), no caffeine, no refined foods, no heavily processed foods, no alcohol, no tobacco, no fruits and vegetables that were not organic, in season, or local. That was the gist of the diet.

Oprah gasped, "Well, what's left?"

"Beans," the lady jokingly said, and Oprah didn't look so happy. The lady spoke about how great the diet makes you feel, how wrinkles fade and excess weight goes down, how you need less sleep and feel better than ever. She was raving about this diet and emphasizing that it was to be maintained only for twenty-one days.

I watched the whole program. I was thinking, "This is pretty good. This is a good diet that she's recommending, and she's on Oprah Winfrey, so millions of people were most likely watching. This diet would affect not only the individual but would have far-reaching consequences in our world, directly affecting the plants, the animals, the water, the earth, and its people."

Every single stage of animal agriculture involves heavy pollution, massive amounts of greenhouse gases, and colossal quantities of energy and waste. Millions of people across the globe are faced with droughts and water shortages. Half of all the water used in the United States is used to raise animals for food. It takes 5,000 gallons of water to produce one pound of meat, while growing one pound of wheat requires only twenty-five gallons. You save more water by not eating a pound of meat than you do by not showering for an entire year.[1] The animals being raised to become food produce 130 times more excrement as the entire U.S. population, roughly 87,000 pounds per second, all without the benefit of waste treatment systems. The Environmental Protection Agency (EPA) reports that chicken, hog, and cattle excrement have polluted 35,000 miles of rivers in twenty-two states and contaminated groundwater in seventeen of them. The EPA states that dangerous fecal bacteria from farm sewage, including E. coli, cause serious illness in humans.[2]

But the author on Oprah's show didn't mention any of that, and I was disappointed. I don't want to be too critical, but if you're on a spiritual path, then your goal is just going to be different from that of the norm. You're not going to be able to stop at "a perfect body." You would have to move way past your own perfect body toward a goal that would include the world in which you live.

* * *

The channels that run within our body are called nadis. Nad means to flow, like the river. In India, the rivers are thought of as holy. There are holidays in India when pilgrims enter on arduous journeys to the rivers in order to collect a small amount of water and bring it home. It is said that, from ancient times, the rivers have washed the feet of the saints, gods, and gurus, and so the water of the rivers have been bowed down to and worshiped. If your house stood by the riverbanks, automatically, in your next life, you would be born to a higher world.

But now in India all the industrial waste is pumped into the rivers, and their sacredness has been forgotten. American factory-farming practices are seeping into Indian culture, and soon the rivers will be even more polluted. In times like these, it is the yogi who reminds the people how to use the rivers without abusing them.

1. John Robbins, *The Food Revolution,* p. 238, 236.
2. Ed Ayres, "Will We Still Eat Meat?" *Time,* 8 November, 1999.

Barley Balls

गुरुर्ब्रह्मा: गुरुर्विष्णुः गुरुर्देवो महेश्वरः ।
गुरुः साक्षात् परंब्रह्म तस्मै श्रीगुरवे नमः ॥

Gurur Brahmāḥ Gurur Vishnuḥ Gurur Devo Mahesvaraḥ
Guruḥ Sāksāt Paraṃ Brahma Tasmai Śrī Gurave Namaḥ

Our creation is that Guru, the duration of our lives is that Guru,
our trials, illnesses, calamities, and the death of our body is that Guru.
There is a Guru that is nearby, and a Guru that is beyond the beyond.
I offer all my efforts to the Guru, the remover of darkness.

—FROM THE *GURU STOTRAM*, A SELECTION FROM *GURU GITA* AS GIVEN IN UTTARAKHAND SECTION OF *SKANDA PURANA*

Once upon a time, there was a young boy in Tibet who was very unruly and mischievous. So his parents thought it would be a good idea to send him to the monastery, where he would get a good training. The young boy went into the monastery and in due course he became a monk. At the monastery, the monks were fed bread made from barley flour, and this young monk would steal scraps of the flour, roll it into little balls, and let the balls become hard. Then he became really good at flicking them at the senior monks as they made their way to morning prayers. So adept was the young monk at flicking them that the other monks couldn't figure out where the barley balls were coming from. When he wasn't flicking the barley balls, the young monk was doing something similar; so he acquired a reputation at the monastery for being disrespectful and causing trouble.

One day, a great abbot came to visit the monastery. As one of the high monks was showing the abbot around the grounds, they came across this young, unruly monk. The high monk introduced the two to each other, and the abbot took a good long look at the young monk, up and down, and then hitting him on the head said,

"You look very good. You look very bright. You are going to go very far. You are a great gift to the monastery." He repeated this and hit the boy on the head several times.

After this experience, the young monk began to study very seriously. He stopped throwing barley balls and became known as a bookworm. It was as if one switch had been turned off and another one turned on—such was the blessing he had received from this abbot. It was as if he had been walking down one road, had left it completely, and was now walking on another, so dramatic was the switch.

Some time passed, and all the monks had to flee Tibet and make the arduous journey into India. Once they had arrived, the monks realized they had left behind several very important texts and none of them had any copies. However, it turned out that this young monk, now a little older, had memorized them, and was able to recite them to the monks, who wrote them down. Thus, on account of him, these texts were saved.

Decades later, now as a man in his eighties, the monk was invited to New Jersey, where he taught many Westerners. He could see that they were good and bright and would go very far and become a gift to the place where they lived.

The abbot who had hit the monk on the head and told him

he was good was the *Guru Sakshat* mentioned in the Sanskrit verse above: the *guru* who is nearby. It's the person who needs to be close enough to hit you on the head, the teacher who makes you stop being unruly. It's the teacher who gets you to stop being engaged in fruitless activities, to stop delaying your spiritual practice and start following those special instincts that we all have.

What the *Guru Sakshat* sees in the student is already there. Goodness and brightness is in everybody in the form of potential. The *guru* nearby sees that potential, and you begin to feel what the *guru* sees. The *guru* is the flipper of the switch.

O Happy Day

योगश्चित्तवृत्तिनिरोधः ॥ २ ॥

yōgāś citta vṛtti nirodhaḥ

Yoga is when the fluctuations of the mind stop.

—MASTER PATANJALI'S *YOGA SUTRAS*, BOOK ONE, SUTRA 2

तस्य वाचकः प्रणवः ॥ २७ ॥

tasya vācakaḥ praṇavaḥ

The expression of Isvara is AUM. At the back of the whole creation is harmony.

—MASTER PATANJALI'S *YOGA SUTRAS*, BOOK ONE, SUTRA 27

The sound of God is AUM. That is something cryptic to ponder. It's like a seed. *Yogash chitta vritti nirodah,* yoga happens or yoga exists when the activity in the mind comes to a standstill.

Once a student of mine came up to me after class. "I really like to meditate," she said.

"That's great," I replied.

My student told me she had moved from California, where she had been living in an isolated place by the sea. When she meditated, there was just herself and the sea, and maybe some birds would perch nearby and sing. My student found that those natural sounds were conducive to her meditation. Now she was living in New York City. She said she heard trucks on the road, horns blowing, neighbors yelling, car alarms, and sirens. She found these noises were not conducive to her meditation.

"What should I do?" she asked. It was a good, sincere, and common question.

Most everything produces sound. The moon and stars and galaxies create sound waves.

I recall once hearing the sound of sleet falling. You could tell by the sound it was neither snow nor rain, but sleet. When the heart beats, it makes a sound. If you become nervous, that sound becomes louder. Yogic breathing is described as sonorous. When the baby emerges from the womb, everyone is waiting to hear a sound. Then the newborn screams, and you know that he or she is alive.

Getting away or separating ourselves from sound is not possible or necessary. What happens often and is normal when we meditate is that we hear sounds and begin to categorize them as good, bad, pleasurable, etc. and feel the need to escape. We try to close it all out, or wait for the day when we can be secluded in a cave, to feel like "Now it's quiet, I can finally meditate."

There's a better way. Suppose I'm talking and you're listening. I can hear your silence and you can hear me talking. In that way, your silence and my sound become connected. You're giving me your silence, I'm giving you my sound, and we're having an exchange. In that exchange is some peace. We're learning how to listen. As soon as we start labeling, we're labeling. We're not listening. Meditation is listening and not labeling. If someone is speaking to you and you're judging him or her or thinking of what you might tell them, then you're not listening. You're somewhere else. Listening is opening up to sound. The sound of God and the sound of others.

When we meditate, we can hear all the different sounds without labeling them as good, bad, pleasurable, etc., and without imposing our judgments, definitions, and reactions. We can be quiet. Master Patanjali says in *The Yoga Sutra* that if we listen to sound without the chitter-chatter of the conditioned mind, free from our labels, if we listen to it as pure sound, then we will hear a symphony. We will hear AUM, the sacred sound in all sounds, the meaning not the explanation. That is why we chant AUM—to speed up the arrival of the happy day when we're no longer harassed by sound, but rather at peace with sound and its greater dimension.

Time Passed

देहिनोऽस्मिन् यथा देहे कौमारं यौवनं जरा ।
तथा देहान्तरप्राप्तिर् धीरस् तत्र न मुह्यति ॥ १३ ॥

dehino'smin yathā dehe kaumāraṃ yauvanaṃ jarā
tathā dehāntaraprāptir dhīras tatra na muhyati

As in the body, the embodied self passes through childhood, youth, and old age,
so is its passage into another body; the wise thereat are not disturbed.

—*THE BHAGAVAD GITA*, CHAPTER TWO, VERSE 13

I have a student named Kelly who is also my friend. Her father was diagnosed with a serious illness, and the doctor said that her father would deteriorate and pass quickly. Kelly decided to rearrange her schedule so that on the weekends she could go with her children to visit her father, who lives in upstate New York. Sometimes, I would see her on Mondays, and she would tell me about her visit.

At first, Kelly told me that her father was in great physical pain and that she had told him that if he could really calm down, he would be able to sense something inside, independent of his physical body, that was not deteriorating. Many people call this the soul. She told him that he should think about this, that it would give him great comfort.

Time passed, and Kelly told her father that he should reflect on his life and think of all the people in his life who had touched him, helped him, or taught him in some way. Before it was too late, he should thank as many people as he could, including those he otherwise might not have thought of. Even if some of these people no longer existed in their physical form, he could communicate with their souls. The gratitude would bring him comfort.

Time passed, and Kelly told her father to think about others who suffer from illnesses also and who are uncomfortable physically, who may be younger than himself, who may be all alone or stranded in a foreign country without speaking the language of their doctors or the people nearby. Many people are in that kind of situation. To the extent that you can think of others in situations like yours, to that extent you won't shrink into smallness. If you are developing compassion, this will bring you great comfort.

Time passed, and Kelly told her father that he should imagine himself in his future life. Even if he didn't believe in one, she said, it would still be a positive activity. He should try to imagine what kind of life he would like. The best life, if he were to come back, would be a life of service, of helping others. Imagine that you will come back a Buddha or a saint, and your presence will relieve others of their suffering.

Time passed, and Kelly told her father that when you die, if you are calm, you could choose to go to celestial spheres where you hear heavenly music. She said that Johann Sebastian Bach spent time in these spheres, and this is where his music comes from. Think about these spheres, she said.

Kelly told me that it seemed to her that her father appreciated and found comfort in all the things she had told him. At the end of his life, she taught him some verses from *The Bhagavad Gita* as well as some Sanskrit words. She told him that the language spoken in heaven is Sanskrit and taught him how to sing to the Lord and not to worry over learning something right before his death. It's never too late to learn anything. Whatever you learn will reverberate in all of your future lives.

Kelly always told me about these visits, and I had a sense that through her poise and strength, her father was able to find peace, that in her atmosphere, he rested. She had the wisdom to know how to spend the last twenty-five weekends with her father. Not only did she have the wisdom, but more importantly, she used the wisdom that she had. If you have wisdom and don't use it, it's of no use.

A Sweet Memory of Jayashree

प्रमाणविपर्ययविकल्पनिद्रास्मृतयः ॥ ६ ॥

pramāṇa viparyaya vikalpa nidrā smṛtayaḥ

Right knowledge, wrong knowledge, imagination, sleep and memory are the five ways that the mind whirls or moves.

—MASTER PATANJALI'S *YOGA SUTRAS,* BOOK ONE, SUTRA 6

One of the movements in the mind is memory, *smritti.* Seeing one thing can remind one of something else. Seeing any old and frail man, always reminds me of my father.

I have a student named Jessica who became a yoga teacher and is doing an apprenticeship with me. One of the things I require of all my apprentices is that they should be able to read and write Sanskrit. I want them to learn the alphabet, how to string the letters together to make words, how to read those words, and how to pronounce them correctly.

I thought Jessica could do all of that. But one day she was about to sing a verse from *The Bhagavad Gita* when she realized she hadn't brought her book. So I offered her mine. Mine had only the Sanskrit, the *devanagari* script, and she couldn't read that. So I said, "Stop. You have to learn the alphabet and be able to string the letters together so that you can read a word. Buckle down and study. Next week I'll quiz you. Just learn the alphabet."

Next week came, and she said, "Oh, I've had a very busy week." She didn't think my quizzing her at this time was such a great idea.

"Okay, I understand," I said. "You've had a busy week. Let's do it next week, but buckle down and study, and next week I'll quiz you."

The next week, I was out of town, but finally we met. I gave Jessica a sutra and asked her to read it. It was painfully slow for her to get one word out, and there seemed to be a lot of guesswork going on. Afterwards I said, "This is a good beginning. I want you to learn the alphabet, so you can be confident. You have to buckle down. There's no alphabet pill you can take."

"Okay," she said.

The following week came and it was better, but only by one tiny increment. I began to be irritable, and I could feel the impatience rising in me. We were sitting next to each other in a small room without windows, and I could hear the impatience in my voice, and I could see it wasn't helping her.

Then, this sweet memory came to me. I've been studying Sanskrit in India with my blessed teacher Jayashree for over fifteen years. What my student's improvement was from week to week was like mine from year to year. One year, I had actually slid backwards. I was sitting with my teacher, and she was writing words for me to read, I was making many mistakes and felt that I was wasting her time.

I apologized to her. "Jayashree, how do you put up with me?" I asked.

"Oh, no, it is not like that," she replied. "You are learning a language; it is very different from your own. It is coming from a different place, from another time; it is very old. It will be difficult for you to learn, it is normal." Then she said, "I am learning

French. I am studying for many years, and like you, I am making very little improvement. It is very slow. It is difficult for you to learn Sanskrit; it is difficult for me to learn French. We are same." Jayashree is one of the greatest living scholars of Sanskrit and Vedic texts in India, and she is telling me with total matter-of-factness, "We are same."

You can make no progress for a long time, and think nothing is happening, but something is happening all along. All of a sudden, you'll take a big leap. That's what she told me. I left that day totally encouraged, and not feeling inadequate or that I was wasting her time.

As soon as this memory came to me, I became like another person with my student. My impatience dropped. I told her she sounded amazing, and I was sincere. I saw the whole thing differently. I saw that it's hard and that she was trying. We each have our own timing and that needs to be honored. I would spoil the process for both of us if I were to become too focused on the result. Remembering how our teachers have encouraged and imbued confidence in us is a good use of memory.

Contrasts and Metaphors

te li ya le ru raama bhakti marga I la la I la nan tat a

How can I be a better devotee? How can I open my heart? Let me cry not for my own disappointments, but because life is large and touching.

—COMPOSED BY TYAAGARAJA (1767–1847), THE CRYING SAINT WHO LONGED FOR THE LORD

Life is full of contrasts and metaphors, parallelisms that help us feel the value of life. Artists have a deep understanding of this. In classical music, a dark movement opens into a celestial movement and you feel the value of the two movements because they co-exist, because they work in a relationship.

Contrasts are found also in literature. In Ian McEwan's novel *On Chesil Beach,* the father tells the son that the problem with the boy's mother is that she is "brain damaged." She was hit while standing on the railway platform by a door that swung out when a train breaked harder than usual. She was "carrying a shopping bag of meager wartime Christmas presents." As the narrator writes: "The heavy metal edge struck Marjorie Mayhew's forehead with sufficient force to fracture her skull and dislocate in an instant her personality, intelligence, and memory. Her coma lasted just under a week." All along the son has known that something is wrong with his mother, but the father feels his son is now at an age when he can explain what is wrong in medical terms. The father is telling his son. They are in the garden, "under the big elm" where the flowers that the boy's mother planted are growing. The son knows the flowers well, and while listening, he is looking at the flowers and admiring them. He knows the popular and the Latin names of the flowers, and is dwelling on their beauty and their names: "orchis, hellebores and the rare summer snowflake." He's remembering his mother planting them in the garden, and simultaneously, he's sort of listening to the bad news about his mother.

These scenes in literature, in sacred texts, and in life, where contrasts and a wide range of emotions coexist, remind us not to become limited or overly emphatic in our responses to the grand scheme of things.

Satkara

तत्र स्थितौ यत्नोऽभ्यासः ॥ १३ ॥

tatra sthitau yatno'bhyāsaḥ

Practice takes steadiness and effort.

—MASTER PATANJALI'S YOGA SUTRAS, BOOK ONE, SUTRA 13

स तु दीर्घ कालनैरन्तर्य सत्कारासेवितो दृढभूमिः ॥ १४ ॥

sa tu dīrgha kāla nairantarya satkārāsevito dṛḍha bhūmiḥ

Practice becomes firmly grounded when well attended to for a long time, without interruption and in all earnestness.

—MASTER PATANJALI'S *YOGA SUTRAS*, BOOK ONE, SUTRA 14

Sat is right and *kara* is to do. There is usually a right way to do something. Satkara expresses a sensitivity that keeps growing more and more refined, so that what you thought was right at one time, you later realize was not.

One summer, I visited my mother in California, and she was suffering from crippling arthritis and couldn't move her right arm. Because she couldn't drive, she asked, "On Sabbath, will you take me to the synagogue?"

"Sure," I responded. "I'd like to go, too."

The synagogue we went to is Orthodox, so the women sit

upstairs. During the service, the rabbi asks the congregation to stand and everyone rises to sing from the prayer book. Then the rabbi tells the congregation they may be seated. At a certain point, the rabbi explains what we've been reading. Everyone sits and sets the prayer book aside.

I sat down and put the book on the ledge in front of me and leaned back to hear what the rabbi had to say. While English and Sanskrit script goes from left to right, Hebrew script goes from right to left. Not being in the habit of handling books written in Hebrew, I put the prayer book down in such a way that the bottom was on top. Without realizing what I had done, I sat back. My mother who was on my left-hand side took her left hand, put it under her right arm, lifted her right arm, and reached for the prayer book, which is heavy. She picked it up turned it so that the top was on top and then slowly put her sore arm back down. It took a while for it to dawn on me what she was doing, but once I understood, I said, "Oh, I'm sorry."

"It's fine," she said. The lady sitting next to her looked relieved that my mother had turned the book over.

That turning of the book right-side-up is *satkara.* It's sensitivity to the placement of the prayer book with the top on top. It's sensitivity that the altar is better when it's clean. It's a feeling that when the teacher sits before you, you wouldn't stretch your feet out toward him or her. It's this kind of attitude that brings a quality of holiness into one's practice that Master Patanjali is saying one will need.

* * *

Abyasa is the effort to still the mind. It is cultivated over a long time, without interruption, with great care and love.

In 2000, Geshe Michael Roach and some of his students entered into a silent retreat for three years, three months, and three days, and he said it wasn't long enough.

People always asked Sri K. Pattabhi Jois, "How long am I going to have to do these practices?"

"Five thousand years," he would answer. He liked that number. "Five thousand years, yes. You take it. No problem."

Nai is without and *antarya* is interruption or between-ness. So *nairantarya* is without interruption. It means that we shouldn't get off the point, or continually go backwards and forwards. If we do, it will mean that we won't go anywhere and we'll pretty much stay on the same level: a little bit forward, a little bit back.

Yoga is a science, and like a science, it is meant to be systematic. You pick up where you left off, and the next day you pick up where you left off, and in that way you go somewhere.

Satkara is with love. You do everything you can to keep your practice clean and uncontaminated, and special. And even though yoga practice is now very popular, which is a very good thing, it is still very sacred, and should always be received it in that way. You should humble yourself, before the yoga practice, your mat, your cushion, your teachers, your text, and your studies: *satkara* with love, devotion, humility, earnestness, and sincerity. You should never be crude, throwing the mat down or pushing the teacher or another student out of the way. If you do, then you have no practice.

The Airline Magazine

शुचौ देशे प्रतिष्ठाप्य स्थिरम् आसनम् आत्मनः ।
नात्युच्छ्रितं नातिनीचं चैलाजिनकुशोत्तरम् ॥ ११ ॥

śucau deśe pratiṣṭhāpya sthiram āsanam ātmanaḥ
nātyucchritaṃ nātinīcaṃ cailājinakuśottaram

To practice yoga, one should go to a secluded place and lay kusa-grass on the ground and then cover it with a deerskin and a soft cloth. The seat should neither be too high nor too low and should be situated in a sacred place.

—*THE BHAGAVAD GITA*, CHAPTER SIX, VERSE 11

In the Fall of 2008, I was on an airplane and didn't have anything to read. So I began to flip through the airline magazine tucked inside the seat pocket in front of me. I spotted an advertisement for a "farm" selling turkeys that you could buy to cook for Thanksgiving. It showed a picture of a cooked turkey, and it said, "Happy Holidays." The ad went on to say that the "farm" had been around for a long time. It included a graph showing that in the early 1980s, the "farm" had killed (it actually said "killed") several thousand turkeys just for Thanksgiving. Then by the end of the decade, it was tens of thousands of turkeys, and by the 1990s it was hundreds of thousands of turkeys. By the year 2000, a million turkeys were killed, and for 2008, millions of turkeys were going to be killed.

The advertisement was supposed to induce you to buy the turkey. The pitch was that this "farm" was the place to buy your turkey because the number of turkeys they were killing was increasing each decade. They were promoting this activity, and they provided a phone number whereby you could order your turkey in time for Thanksgiving. I read the advertisement several times. At first, I thought I was reading it incorrectly, but then realized I wasn't, and I found it frightening.

Before leaving for my weeklong trip, I had received twenty bouquets of flowers from friends who came to a party I had given. When I returned home, I discovered that nobody had attended to the flowers while I was away, so they didn't look very strong. I sensed, however, there was still some life left in them, so I took the flowers out of the vases, changed the water, and put a little sugar in it, because flowers like sugar. I disposed of the ones that were unsalvageable, and with those that were I pulled off the dead leaves, cut all the stems, and put the flowers back in their vases. In ten minutes, they came back to life. They looked pretty and welcoming and vivid. They had gone from drooping to standing up.

I began to think about those turkeys. We kill with such nonchalance; we make it sound so easy; and the numbers are huge, in the billions. Such killing amounts to an enormous amount of violence in the atmosphere. I was looking at the flowers, bright and beautiful. It became difficult for me to think about the turkeys. That's why I sometimes find it hard as a teacher to speak about vegetarianism, because it's a heavy subject. Billions of animals are discarded.

In this verse from *The Bhagavad Gita,* Lord Krishna tells Arjuna what the best seat for meditation would be. "Get a piece of animal skin," he says, "and sit on that." At the time their conversation took place, there were many more animals in the forest than today, and many fewer people on earth. Yogis felt great reverence, respect, and awe for animals and aspired to acquire some of the great qualities they saw in them. They would sometimes go into the forest, and if they came upon an animal that had died from natural causes, then the yogis, because they wished for something of the attitude of the animal, would tear a fingernail-size piece of the skin off, to put underneath their meditation cushion. Before tearing off that tiny piece of skin, the yogis would make sure that the animal hadn't been punctured in any way. At that time, people hunted with bows and arrows. If the animal had died from human violence, then even if the yogi himself had not killed that animal, the skin could not be used. The yogi could not sit in meditation on the skin of an animal that had been killed by a human being.

A week before Thanksgiving, I was talking to my friend Andrea over the telephone. She was in tears over the number of people coming out of the supermarket with turkeys. She's a sensitive, gentle creature and was almost inconsolable. She wanted to bring those turkeys back to life. The freedom to think like that is great. To question an advertisement that boasts of mass killings brings a sense of freedom for which I'm very grateful. My teachers have taught me to question the things that everyone does without questioning, as opposed to living with nonchalance.

Isis and the Yogi Take Forms

The Goddess Isis was the great and beneficent goddess and mother, whose influence and love pervaded all heaven and Earth and the abode of the dead. She was the personification of the great feminine creative power, which conceived and brought forth every living creature from the gods in heaven to man on the Earth, including the insect on the ground. What she brought forth, she protected and cared for and fed, and nourished and she employed her life in using her power graciously and successfully, not only in creating new beings, but in restoring those that were dead. She was, besides these things, the highest type of a faithful and loving wife and mother and it was in this capacity that the Egyptians honored and worshiped her most. Among her general titles maybe mentioned those of: The Divine One, the Only One, Opener of the Year, Lady of the New Year, Maker of the Sunrise, Lady of Heaven, The Light Giver of Heaven, Lady of the North Wind, Queen of the Earth, Most Mighty One, Queen of the South, Lady of the Solid Earth, Lady of Warmth and Fire, Benefactress, Godmother, Mother of Gold, Lady of Life, Lady of Green Crops, The Green Goddess, Lady of Bread, Lady of Beer, Lady of Abundance, Lady of Joy, Lady of Gladness, Lady of Love, The Maker of Kings, Lady of the Great House, Lady of the House of Fire, the Beautiful Goddess, the Lady of Words of Power, the Wife of the Lord.

—E. A. WALLACE BUDGE, THE GODS OF THE EGYPTIANS

Isis was worshipped as the greatest goddess because she united with all the forms and took on the qualities of all the creatures from the insect to the king. Similarly, the yogi assumes all the forms of all the creatures in the world, from the insect to the king. In yoga practice, these forms are called *asanas.*

We take the form of serpents and birds: *shalabasana,* the locust; *bhujangasana,* the snake; *nakcrasana,* the crocodile; *matseyasana,* the fish; *krounchasana,* the heron; *bhakasana,* the crow; *mayurasana,* the peacock; *ghurudasana,* the eagle; and *rajakapotasana* the pigeon.

We take the form of four-legged animals: *svanasana,* the dog; *gomukasana,* the cow; *ustrasana,* the camel; *simhasana,* the lion; *kurmasana,* the turtle; and *bhekasana,* the frog.

We take the form of the plants: *vrksasana,* the tree; *padmasana,* the flower; and *tadasana,* the mountain.

We take the form of various tools: navasana, the boat; konasana, the compass; halasana, the plow; and dhanurasana, the bow.

We take the form of man: *Virabhadrasana,* the warrior; *Virasana,* the hero; *Hanumanasana,* the savior; *Marichyasana,* the sage; *Vacchistasana,* the saint; *Savasana,* the corpse; *Surya Namaskar,* the sun worshiper; *Chandra Namaskar,* the moon worshiper; *Tara namaskar,* the star worshiper; and *Natarajasana,* dancing Shiva, the Lord himself.

In adopting these poses, yogis assume all the forms of all the creatures in the world, training our minds never to despise any creature. The same universal spirit breathes through all the creatures, from the insect to the king. The yogi becomes the friend to all, the nurturer to all, the protector to all, and can commune and live harmoniously with all. That is yoga. Yoga means to join.

Trust

अज्ञश्चाश्रद्दधानश्च संशयात्मा विनश्यति ।
नायं लोकोऽस्ति न परो न सुखं संशयात्मनः ॥ ४० ॥

ajñaścāśraddadhānaśca saṃśayātmā vinaśyati
nāyaṃ loko'sti na paro na sukhaṃ saṃśayātmanaḥ

The ignorant, the man lacking in devotion, the doubt-filled man, ultimately perishes. The unsettled individual has neither this world (earthly happiness), nor the next (astral happiness), nor the supreme happiness of God.

—*THE BHAGAVAD GITA*, CHAPTER FOUR, VERSE 40

In the early 1990s, my guru in India Sri K. Pattabhi Jois began to have many students who gave him and his family gifts. Often, the gifts were monetary, and in response, my teacher created a trust so there would be a place for the money to be used for charitable projects. Years passed after the trust had been established. Since the family had said nothing further about it, a few students were wondering what the money was being used for, and if it was being used well.

An American woman named Nancy lives in the same town as did my late teacher and is dedicated to a life of service. The Jois family had chosen her to act as the head of the trust. She researches and oversees all the projects and handles all the money. She heard that some students had become skeptical, so she approached the family and said, "In the West, when people give money to non-profit organizations, every three or four months a newsletter is sent out, which shows how much money was collected, and a breakdown is given of how it was spent. With your permission, I would send out such a newsletter."

Guruji was confused. He said that in the scriptures it says that when you give, you should not publicize it. If you publicize it, it automatically becomes something that you do for the sake of your name, and the power of the gift will be greatly diminished. So he did not care for this idea. Nancy continued to try to persuade him, and the last I heard, the family was thinking about it.

The relationship that one has with one's guru or teacher is based on trust, not on suspicion. It is a relationship that's based on faith not doubt, one that needs no external proof. That is the beauty of it.

A great tool that the teacher uses is words. But the teaching itself is much greater than the words and the teacher. If the student is listening to the teacher and understanding the words, but has doubt about the teacher, then that doubt creates a wall between themselves and the essence of the teaching. If the student doesn't quite understand the words that the teacher is using—perhaps the teacher speaks with a thick accent or uses a great deal of Sanskrit—but the student has faith in the teacher, then the deep and vital points of the teaching will be transmitted to the student. The faith that the student places in the teacher opens the door.

Each time we recite a verse like this one from *The Bhagavad Gita,* we are praying that our faith shall increase, so that we can stop doubting life; our circumstances, our teachers, and ourselves minimize our anxiety, and have a basic trust. Even in subject areas that make us uncomfortable, we should have some faith that they're there to propel us to spiritual heights and an unfolding of our essence, our true nature. Everybody has a little bit of faith in something. Some people have faith in what their parents have told them, some don't. Some people have faith in their religion, some don't. Some people have faith in their government, some don't.

The yoga tradition is to have faith in the guru whom we wish to learn from. That faith in and of itself makes us teachable.

Holy Presence

यं हि न व्यथयन्त्येते पुरुषं पुरुषर्षभ ।
समदुःखसुखं धीरं सोऽमृतत्वाय कल्पते ॥ १५ ॥

yaṃ hi na vyathayantyete puruṣaṃ puruṣarṣabha
samaduḥkhasukhaṃ dhīraṃ so'mṛtatvāya kalpate

He who cannot be ruffled by contacts of the senses with their objects,
who is calm and even-minded during pain and pleasure,
he alone is fit to attain everlastingness.

—*THE BHAGAVAD GITA*, CHAPTER TWO, VERSE 15

It's always good, if we can, to settle down. If we do something without first settling down and we botch it up, we may think afterwards, "If only I'd settled down beforehand." It's an important skill to know how to settle down. As a teacher, I've realized that though I may have something inspiring to share, a story or a piece of music, being calm and settled is worth so much to people.

Things change. Sometimes we welcome the change, other times we don't. In any case, life is always on the move. Because life is in flux, seekers—from ancient times up to the present day—have wondered, "Is there something that does not change? That was, is, and will always be?" The sages and poets have pondered this question. They thought that if there were something unchanging and undying, it would help people to get through the ups and downs in life.

Several years ago, I was fortunate enough to see the Dalai Lama giving teachings in New York. My husband and I were sitting in the theatre where the teachings were to take place, and it was very crowded. A lady appeared onstage and told us that His Holiness was delayed, and asked us to please be patient; when she knew more, she said, she would tell us. It turned out that many of the people in the audience knew each other. Many of them were monks, and it was like a reunion. Someone on the second floor would spot a friend down below in the orchestra section and begin waving and yelling "hello." It was noisy, there was a lot of commotion, and it was wild in the theatre.

Finally, the lady returned to the stage and announced that His Holiness had arrived and that within a few minutes he would begin his program. In three seconds, a hush of silence came over the whole auditorium. Quickly, efficiently, orderly, and gracefully, those who had left their seats tiptoed back to them. You could hear the quiet, and you could feel the presence of something holy nearby.

A week after this event, I attended teachings on *The Hatha Yoga Pradipika,* given by Geshe Michael Roach. The teachings continued until midnight, which means that I didn't arrive home until one o'clock in the morning, when I'm usually asleep. However, even though I returned home so late, I couldn't fall asleep right away. I couldn't wake my husband because he's a nurse and has to get up at five in the morning.

I had recently found out that American soldiers who had been in Iraq and Afghanistan and were wounded badly were now hospitalized in Germany. The hospital had a shortage of blankets, and the soldiers were cold. An organization had been formed for people to knit blankets and send them over. Several thousand of these blankets had been made. When I found myself unable to sleep or after arriving home late at night, I would knit for an hour. This is what I did that night. I tiptoed around the apartment and kept on only one tiny lamp to knit under. Sitting there, quietly knitting a blanket, almost in the dark, I felt the presence of something holy nearby.

The masters tell us that the presence of something holy is in and around us everywhere and all the time. The reason we miss it is because we're too caught up in the ups and downs and changes that occur in our lives. Because we miss the holy presence, there's a shadow of doubt, a feeling that something is not quite right, even in the happiest of moments, which causes a great deal of agitation and often leads to violence.

So it's crucial to re-establish our connection to the holy presence continuously. That is what spiritual practices are for, to tap into what is unchanging and eternal. When we go deep into our practices, whatever they may be—meditation, *asanas,* a vegan diet, knitting blankets, or being a nurse—the more we will feel the holy presence in our life, and the less imprisoned we feel by the ups and downs.

The Fabulous Mr. Roth

गुरुर्ब्रह्माः गुरुर्विष्णुः गुरुर्देवो महेश्वरः ।
गुरुः साक्षात् परंब्रह्म तस्मै श्रीगुरवे नमः ॥

Gurur Brahmāḥ Gurur Vishnuḥ Gurur Devo Mahesvaraḥ
Guruḥ Sāksāt Paraṃ Brahma Tasmai Śrī Gurave Namaḥ

Our creation is that Guru, the duration of our lives is that Guru,
our trials, illnesses, calamities, and the death of our body is that Guru.
There is a Guru that is nearby, and a Guru that is beyond the beyond.
I offer all my efforts to the Guru, the remover of darkness.

—FROM THE *GURU STOTRAM*, A SELECTION FROM *GURU GITA* AS GIVEN IN UTTARAKHAND SECTION OF *SKANDA PURANA*

There is an American writer named Philip Roth. In his book *Patrimony*, he describes to the reader how he told his father not to include him in the will that his father was making. He thought it best for his portion to be divided amongst his brothers who were struggling raising children and had not had the financial success that he had experienced. Without any argument, the father said, "Okay."

Time passed, and the father developed a terrible cancer and became ill. Because the brothers were working to make ends meet, Roth took it upon himself to look after his father, which involved doing things that most people would find unpleasant: such as cleaning up what his father had thrown up, bathing him against his own will, and putting up with his chronic irritability.

During this difficult time, Roth began to reconsider the father's will. He felt now that all the children should have an equal portion of what his father might leave to them and regretted that he had relinquished his share. However, he thought that if he told his family of his change of heart, with his father in such a condition, it would upset everyone. So he decided to live with it.

Time passed, and Roth took his father to the doctor. The doctor had told his father that if he had any questions, he should write them down and bring them to the appointment. On that particular day, the father had some questions written on a little yellow post-it that he had folded several times. He reached into his pocket and took out this tiny piece of paper, unfolded it, and asked the doctor, "How much longer will I live? What is the best I can expect? What is the worst I can expect? Will I ever be able to have sex again?"

The doctor answered these questions. Then the old man took the post-it, folded it again several times, and put it back into his pocket. When they were driving home, Roth thought to himself: "You know what? It's fine. I don't want my portion. But I do want that piece of paper that's in my father's pocket. If I could just have that, it will be okay."

Cherishing our parents in thought and deed and taking care of them is a way of serving God, in the form of our parents. After Roth was able to transcend the illness, the nausea, the smells, the irritability, and the will, he realized that it was his father's life itself that he cherished.

In this verse, Guru Brahma is honoring the teacher in the form of our birth, the circumstances, the seed and the egg, and those who raise us. Because of all that, we are given a body, and that body supports an auspicious life, from which we can progress as human beings.

Manhattan Skyline

वस्तु साम्ये चित्त भेदात् तयोर्विभक्तः पन्थाः ॥ १५ ॥

vastu sāmye citta-bhedāt tayor vibhaktaḥ panthāḥ

When the object is the same, but the mental field is different, the way of perceiving or the level of understanding the object will be different.

—MASTER PATANJALI'S *YOGA SUTRAS*, BOOK FOUR, SUTRA 15

The studio I rent for my work occupies a corner of the building. It has windows on two walls and because it's on the corner, those views are very different from each other. One is of the Manhattan skyline, a beautiful view. When I was in Egypt, I told the owner of my hotel that I thought the pyramids were stunning. He said, "But you have the Manhattan skyline!"

The other windows face a row of modest Brooklyn houses that have back yards with picnic tables and clotheslines with laundry hanging from them. I like having such different views of the same city. It helps to remind me that there are many ways of looking at things and many different vantage points, depending on the view. That is why people don't always see the same thing. We should keep this in mind, especially when we are critical and judgmental of others. How we see everything depends on our viewpoint.

I've been a yoga teacher for a fairly long time, and I used to have students whose behavior bothered me. They would talk while

I was talking, stretch and indulge in neck rolls, rummage through bags, and arrive late to class. I would think it was rude and inappropriate.

I would also have students who kept doing things slightly differently from each instruction I gave. I would think, "What's with that?" I had very clearly stated what to do. Or a student would leave early, and I'd be saying to myself, "But it's not over yet!" Or someone would leave during meditation, make a racket while everybody was trying to be quiet, and I would look to see who it was. I would be troubled by a bad feeling toward that student. "Can't they see that everybody else is trying to be quiet?" I would think. "Why are they disturbing everybody?" I would judge and build up an attitude. Judging others, feeling that they don't attempt to reach your standard, and then dismissing them—all these create a lot of barriers.

As the years have passed, my view has changed. When a student is lying down while I am talking, I'll think, "They must be tired." Life is tiring. Aren't you sometimes a little tired? I mean, *I'm tired.* I'm happy that the student can have a place to lie down since she must have been tired. When someone left my class early one day, but had hung in for a whole hour before leaving, I thought to myself, "Wow! it's great to make it through two-thirds of a yoga class." When a student was making a great deal of noise during meditation, I thought, "This student is agitated." As human beings, until we're enlightened, we're going to be agitated. I was happy that that person was here, and I hoped that all the calm energy in the room could help this person have a moment of relief.

I see this softening in myself, and I rejoice. I'm very happy that I don't quickly decide I don't like the way someone looks or what someone is doing or saying or thinking or drinking. At whom do you look when you are looking at somebody, and from where are you looking? If we look at each other and see the complexities, struggles, and all the angles, and take it all in when we look at the faces of everyone in the world, we will find something just right that is as it is.

With all that said, I still think students should be encouraged not to leave class early. Staying power is a beautiful thing on the mat, on the meditation cushion, and on the spiritual path. But staying power is difficult to develop. We always want to be somewhere other than where we are. A yoga class is a good opportunity to change that pattern by maintaining the absence of desire to go anywhere else for the duration of the yoga class. In any case, now, if I see a number of students slipping out early, I ask myself what am I doing to see this in my world? What is my part in it?

Saucha

शौचसंतोषतपःस्वाध्यायेश्वरप्रणिधानानि नियमाः ॥ ३२ ॥

śaucha saṃtoṣa tapaḥ svādhyāyeśvara praṇidhānāni niyamāḥ

Cleanliness, contentment, self-discipline, Self-study, devotion to God. These are the five observances.

—MASTER PATANJALI'S *YOGA SUTRAS*, BOOK TWO, SUTRA 32

Saucha means to be clean, radiant, and brilliant, inside and out.

I had a cat named Nellie. When she was three-and-a-half years old she swallowed a whole clove of garlic, which got stuck in her small intestine and obstructed her breathing. We took her to the hospital. The surgeons operated on her to remove the obstruction and told us the surgery went well, and we could pick our cat up in two days. However, two days later, Nellie was stricken with pneumonia. The veterinarians kept her in a cage with oxygen and assured us that in two days she would be better. Two days later, her breathing was better, but her wound had become infected. For two weeks, this went on; one thing got better, but a new problem arose. Finally, we could see that all of this was too much for the little one, and we understood that we would have to let her go.

Everyone at the hospital agreed that Nellie was the sweetest cat ever. The vets marveled that not once had she become irritated. My husband and I were with her in the last hour of her life. In one corner of her cage was a cushion on which she was resting. At one point she got up and walked to the opposite corner of the cage, where her litter box stood, and peed. Then, she walked back to her cushion and died. She died clean. The doctors said it was remarkable that as sick as she was, she didn't simply pee in her bed. They said she had great dignity.

That is *saucha*—the privilege of keeping yourself, your surroundings, and your world clean.

Nothing Belongs to Us

अस्तेयप्रतिष्ठायां सर्वरत्नोपस्थानम् ॥ ३७ ॥

asteya pratiṣṭhāyāṃ sarva ratnopasthānam

When one is established in non-stealing, one develops an awareness of the jewels nearby.

—MASTER PATANJALI'S *YOGA SUTRAS*, BOOK TWO, SUTRA 37

If we want to attain *Samàdhi,* to stop seeing only differences, to stop being miserable and bringing others into our misery, then we need a path. We are all much more than we seem and we sense that; but in order to realize it, we need direction. So Master Patanjali gives us a clear path.

The first step on the path is *yama. Yama* is a vow (*vratam*) to not hurt others in thought, word, or deed, but to uplift them and take care of them. That is the beginning of the path. *Samadhi* is the end of the path, where you're set down in sameness, implying that you don't live in a world of others. Those are the bookends of the path. Even though the yogi doesn't wear robes, we have vows. *Yama* is made up of five parts. The second part is *asteya*: not stealing.

My landlady's mother in India loves chocolate. She always tells me, "There's no good chocolate in India. Where you come from there is good chocolate." So, whenever I go to India, I bring her chocolate. I can be frugal when it comes to certain things, and extravagant when it comes to others. I tend to be extravagant when it comes to bringing her chocolate. It's a big project. I gather many different bars of chocolate from many different regions.

When I get to India, I go upstairs to my room and settle in. Then I open my suitcase, find the chocolate, and go downstairs to look for Tara, the grandmother, the queen of the house, who is always in the kitchen.

"Tara?" I ask.

"Yes!"

"I have something for you."

"Yes, wait one minute," Tara says. She washes her hands, because she's always making food, and wipes them on her nightgown, because she's always in her nightgown. Then she shuffles out of the kitchen.

"Take your seat," she says.

We sit at the table.

"Give it here!" she orders, and she takes it all. "Yes, yes, you have brought chocolate. Very good." Then she examines it all carefully, saying, "O nuts! O dark! Ooo Switzerland chocolate!" Then she says, "Wait one minute." She takes all of it into the kitchen, opens up every bar, cuts a small piece from each bar and puts them on a plate. Then she cuts some pieces of mango or pineapple to embellish the plate, and returns to the table. She places it down underneath my nose, and says, "Here. Eat chocolate." The very first thing she does with my offering, is offer it back.

That's *asteya*. Offering back everything that you've been given. It's the opposite of feeling entitled to things. It's the sense that nothing is yours. Everything is on loan—even your body, even your mind. Everything should be taken care of nicely and given back. Nothing is yours; you're not entitled to anything. This is difficult, because if you've paid for something you start to feel entitled. The idea that you've stolen that thing that you've paid for is dismissed, because you think, "Well I paid for it." But if you pay for milk (organic or not), you've still stolen it from the cow. Just because you pay for it doesn't entitle you to the milk of another species. If you buy six acres of land with a pond and a little house, buying that land does not entitle you to chop down the trees on that land. *Asteya* is the sense that things are not yours to take. There are ancient Vedic prayers that ask God to protect us from thinking things are ours. Knowing that we're not entitled to take as much of, and whatever we want, makes life precious.

If you are firmly established (*pratistayam*) in each one of those yamas, there is a fruit. When one stops stealing from others, all (*sarva*) the jewels (*ratno*) steadily come (*upastanam*). My husband and I never lock anything up: our house, our car, are left open. We don't even know where our house keys are. Even when we lived in New York City, we always left our apartment door open and our car unlocked. Sometimes people would go into the apartment or the car and we would find things, like traces. Someone would leave a piece of vegan chocolate cake in my car or refrigerator, or a bouquet of flowers on my kitchen table. Once this antique Chinese vase from the Ming Dynasty appeared in our house. If you don't take things that aren't yours, you'll never have to worry about things: they'll come miraculously.

For Asako

मैत्रियादिषु बलानि ॥ २३ ॥

maitriyādiṣu balāni

Strength arises out of compassion.

—MASTER PATANJALI'S *YOGA SUTRAS*, BOOK THREE, SUTRA 24

Maitri is love, friendship, and compassion. *Balani* is strength. This word appears often in *The Bhagavad Gita* in reference to Arjuna's arms. Where does strength come from? Master Patanjali says it comes from friendship.

On one occasion, I was giving a lecture and some of my friends came. This gave me strength. Someone left a drink made with fermented tea, or kombucha, at my seat. The drink advertises that it boosts the immune system, aids digestion, brings about healthy skin and hair, and reverses aging. The drink would give me some strength; but, because my friend put it there, it would give me even more.

I once had a friend who was Japanese named Asako, who from our first meeting I felt very close to. She was beautiful and had been a dancer, but cancer destroyed her body. She became very sick, underwent continuous chemotherapy, and became emaciated. She handled all of this with grace and equanimity and never complained. Then she lost all of her long, black hair. She telephoned me, and it touched me that she called to tell me about her hair, for we didn't speak too often. She told me that this was now too much, that she was broken and couldn't go on any longer. I didn't know what to say. I just listened and said I would come visit soon. After we spoke, I thought to myself that I should cut my hair. I didn't have long beautiful black hair—it was straggly and ordinary, and of medium length. "But," I thought, "If she can't have hers, then I don't want mine, so I'll just quietly cut it off."

When I cut it, I felt very strong afterwards. My action expressed the solidarity between Asako and me. It gave both of us strength. Then my friend passed away, and I've been thinking that I should grow my hair again. However, I'm not quite ready, because the absence of my hair reminds me of this friendship.

In our lives, we will have many friends. The yogi is described as friend to all, including the plants and animals. The Buddha said, "The next time I come into the world, my name will be Maitreya." Friendship can be expressed in a myriad of ways. Each time we express friendship, we become strong. Strength accumulates. It accumulates to such a degree that one person could uplift the whole world.

Sweeping the Dust

Sometimes we may sing a verse from a holy ancient text, and we may not know what it "means." For years, I sang prayers in my Sanskrit class in India without knowing their meaning. If I asked, my teachers Jayashree and Narasimhan would quickly tell me that I would not understand it anyway, and then Jayashree would say, "Let us sing." This went on for years.

In India, traditionally the student would be called upon to recite a whole text by heart before being introduced to any discussion of its meaning. My teachers always assured me that not knowing the meaning was not something I should worry about. There is a meaning that you can go out and get, it's almost like shopping. Like so much in life, that meaning is information that you accumulate and fill your mind with. But there is another meaning that the teacher desires for his student. This is the meaning that comes to the student from inside.

Life is like this. You may sweep the floor, and the meaning—the functional purpose—is to remove the dust. But while you are sweeping, the meaning of the ceremony of beautifying your life may push through the surface of what seems to be a chore. You may like to eat on the floor (people all over the world do), even if you have tables and chairs. You may think it is simply more comfortable. But while sitting on the floor you might suddenly appreciate the meaning of sitting low on the ground, connected to the earth that yields your food.

Asana practice—the yoga exercises of posture—is all about this. You lock your anus, pull the belly in and up, lift the chest, drop the shoulders, and lengthen the neck, so that you can breathe properly. This has a physical meaning as well as a meaning connected to safety. But halfway through practice, another meaning comes to you, and that is what makes the practice meaningful. That meaning may not present itself in the form of a concept. It will be broader, because we are all broader than our concepts. That meaning cannot be defined, but it can be felt. Meaning is healing; it comes to us in time. Meaning shines through us; it has an aura. It connects us to our spirit and teaches us to be good people.

The Guru's Feet

सप्तसागरपर्यन्तं तीर्थस्नानफलं तु यत्।
गुरुपादपयोबिन्दोः सहस्रांशेन तत्फलम् ॥ ४५ ॥

saptasāgaraparyantaṃ tīrthasnānaphalaṃ tu yat
gurupādapayobindoḥ sahasrāṃśena tat phalaṃ

Whatever merit is acquired by one, through pilgrimages and from bathing in the sacred waters, extending to the seven seas, cannot be equal to even one thousandth part of the merit derived from partaking of the water with which the guru's feet are washed.

—FROM THE *GURU GITA*, VERSE 45

The manipura chakra is located behind the solar plexus and is connected to the sense of sight. Eye exercises are said to be beneficial for this chakra. In the *Yoga Sutras*, Master Patanjali says that we don't see correctly. Our vision is conditioned, and therefore distorted, contaminated, and simplistic. If we want to improve our vision, we will need more than eyeglasses.

In order to see correctly, we need a mind that is not strained with conflict, fragmentation, and twirling. Then we will be able to see what the enlightened beings see when they see all sentient beings. In *The Hatha Yoga Pradipika*, Yogi Swatmarama says that to steady the mind it is helpful to look at things that are calming, like a flame on a candle.

Let's say you organize your drawer. You take everything out, get rid of all the stuff you don't need, and neatly put back what is left. Later, when you open up the drawer, you think "Ah! Order." You enjoy a general sense that things are in order in and beyond your drawers. When you see the space you have created, that vision reminds you that what you can't see is more important than what you can.

A student of mine is a disciple of Mata Amritanandamayi Ma, also known as Ammachi, the great hugging saint in India. My student was asked to wash Ammachi's feet. When my student was done, she asked if it would be all right for her to keep the water. "Yes, keep it!" Ammachi said. My student poured the water into a glass bottle, wrapped up the bottle, placed a bow on it, and gave it to me.

I placed the bottle on my altar, where I look at it frequently. When I do, I see the student's love for me, and see that she appreciates me. I see 72,000 lifetimes of good deeds that she must have performed to attain the place where she is washing the saint's feet. I see the saint's reflection in the water. I see the lineage in the Eastern traditions that honors the feet of the guru to the extent that devotees wash them. (In India, you see pictures of saints' feet everywhere you go.) When you bow to the guru, it is always to touch his feet in a gesture of humility.

In essence, what I see is beyond the name and form of the bottle of water. But it is helpful to be able to touch the object. What I see opens the door to something that can't be seen. If the door weren't ever opened, I'd begin to die.

Rainbow Falafel

ॐ द्यौः शान्तिः अन्तरिक्ष शान्तिः
पृथिवी शान्तिरापः शान्तिरोषधयः शान्तिः ।
वनस्पतयः शान्तिर्विश्वेदेवाः शान्तिर्ब्रह्म शान्तिः
सर्वं शान्तिः शान्तिरेव शान्तिः सा मा शान्तिरेधि ॥
ॐ शान्तिः शान्तिः शान्तिः ॐ

oṃ dyauḥ śāntiḥ antarikṣaṃ śāntiḥ
pṛthivī śāntir āpaḥ śāntir oṣadhayaḥ śāntiḥ
vanaspatayaḥ śāntir viśve devāḥ śāntir
brahma śāntiḥ sarvaṃ śāntiḥ śāntir eva śāntiḥ sā mā śāntir edhi
oṃ śāntiḥ śāntiḥ śāntiḥ oṃ

May the heavens: the sun, moon, stars, galaxies, and all zodiac signs be in peace and harmony. May the space between the earth and the sun, moon, and stars be peaceful and without pollution. May our mother earth be happy and peaceful and free from all pollution. May all the waters be peaceful and free from pollution—the oceans, rivers, dinking water, and rain, with no acid rain. May all the medicinal herbs and plants be in their natural state and be free from pollution. May the whole vegetable kingdom, especially all trees and forests, be in a natural state, healthy and free from disease due to pollution. May all the elements—earth, water, fire, air, and ether—and all the cosmic forces be in peace and harmony, without pollution. May our body, mind, and soul and all of existence be in peace and harmony, free from pollution. May everything, in and out, be peaceful and in natural harmony, without pollution. May peace itself be real peace, not artificially maintained by military and police forces or balance of nuclear power. And last but not least, may that natural peace, harmony, and unity blossom and flourish through us. AUM Shanthi Shanthi Shanthi: peace—physically, mentally, and spiritually.

—FROM *THE VEDAS*, TRANSLATION AND COMMENTARY BY SHRI BRAHMANANDA SARASWATI

One of the favorite aspects of my job is that, on any given day, my students come from all over the world. I have had people in my class from Brazil, Russia, Venezuela, Argentina, Colombia, Costa Rica, Mexico, every state in the United States, Vancouver and other Canadian cities, England, Germany, France, Italy, Spain, Madrid, Turkey, Iran, Lebanon, Israel, Kuwait, Guam, Indonesia, Afghanistan, India, China, Japan, The Philippines, South Africa, Latvia, Senegal, and Albania. These people have told me about their native places, so when I read the newspaper or hear the news, I feel concerned about what's going on there. Since I have not visited all of these locations, the faces of my students help my imagination enter their places.

I have a dear student and friend named Rima, who is also a yoga teacher. She comes from Lebanon but now lives in New York. Her country has been subjected to instability and violence for many years. She grew up in this atmosphere. A few years ago, a revered and popular Lebanese government official was assassinated, and it was believed that the Syrian government had something to do with this political murder. My friend was very upset. She telephoned me, crying. "What am I going to do?" she asked, over and over again. Because she is here and her family and friends are in Lebanon, she felt helpless. So I listened.

The day and evening passed and I wanted to call her back to see how she was doing.

"How do you feel?" I asked.

"Much better," she replied.

"What did you do?"

"There is a Syrian restaurant on Seventeenth Street called Rainbow Falafel," Rima said. "It's a little hole-in-the-wall. I like the Syrian people who run the restaurant. I went there and hung out with the owners. We shared in our heartache and I ate a falafel."

After Rima left the restaurant, she went to teach her yoga class. She told the class about the situation in her country, and about having gone to eat a falafel and hang out with the Syrian owners. A Jewish student in her class was very moved by what my friend Rima said. The next day, the student called Rima and said, "I want to go to this Syrian restaurant and have a falafel. Could you please tell me exactly where it is and if there is any specific way you like to have your falafel prepared? I want to know because I want my falafel to be exactly how yours was. I want the exact same falafel."

So my friend told me this story. It's a blessing to have people like this in our community because communities need leaders.

My friend's response to the situation was, "What am I going to do?" What she came up with was to share food with her so-called enemies. To act on that kind of fine impulse does not happen overnight. The spiritual path on which her feet are firmly planted has led her to that impulse. She has clearly done the work. This work, which cannot be skipped, is called *sadhana* in Sanskrit. It means to give oneself over to reaching one's potential. The student who wants the falafel to taste exactly like the teacher's is dear to my heart. She embraces lineage. It's called *sruti parampara* in Sanskrit. When things of value are handed down, one wishes to treat and experience them *exactly* as they were handed down.

If your heart aches when you hear about an earthquake in Haiti or floods in Sri Lanka, it is called being awake, or *bodhi chitta* in Sanskrit.

Yoga Communities

A few years ago, I had a student who had been coming to class regularly for several years. She wanted to make a change and practice early in the morning in order to be at work by nine. I don't teach before nine. My student was very athletic, liked to windsurf, ski, and rock-climb. She was looking for a practice that would be rigorous and asked me where she should go. I knew of a place where she would be finished by 8:30. It would meet her requirements for rigor, and the teacher who runs that school is a dear friend of mine.

My student went to this place and said to this teacher, "I'd like to be your student. I'm Ruth's student."

He said, "If you're Ruth's student, then you can't be my student, and if you want to be my student, you can't be Ruth's student."

She said, "I'll get back to you."

She left upset. She just hadn't expected the meeting to go this way. She telephoned me and asked whether she could see me. We got together and she relayed what had happened. I was calm. "There's nothing to be upset about," I said. "He's a dedicated teacher with an exceptional school, you'll be out by 8:30, and it is rigorous. Why don't you just follow his instructions and become his student?"

"All right," she said. Several years have passed and she remains happily his student.

I had another student who wanted to make a change and practice early in the morning in order to be at work by nine. She, too, was looking for a practice that would be rigorous and asked me where she should go. I recommended the same place. She went and said to this same teacher, "I'd like to be your student. I'm Ruth's student." He lit up and smiled. He was very warm and said, "Please say *hello* to Ruth for me and come tomorrow morning at six a.m. for class."

It makes me happy that someone who works at another yoga center feels affection and respect for someone who works at a different yoga center. It's sad when that doesn't occur. I'm hopeful that the boundaries between yoga schools will diminish and the positive effect that the communities have on the world will keep increasing.

So much good is coming out of these communities. Shiva Rea has a project for planting trees in places that have been devastated from fires. Seane Corn started YouthAids. My friend Courtney McDowell, with great support from Eddie Stern of Ashtanga Yoga Shala NY, and Barbara Verrochi and Kristin Leigh of The Shala, established Bent on Learning to teach yoga to kids in public schools. My best friend, Lisa Schrempp, goes on her own into prisons and teaches yoga to people on death row. My spiritual sister, Yogeswari, works tirelessly, has created Azahar Foundation, and teaches yoga in all corners of the world, wherever terrible things are happening specifically as a result of war. She's totally unafraid, and such an inspiration! She carries a library of books and a harmonium everywhere she travels.

My guru, Sri K. Pattabhi Jois, created the Jois Charitable Trust to raise funds for those afflicted with extreme hardships, to protect the forests, and to encourage and maintain the ethical treatment of animals in India.

My teachers, David Life and Sharon Gannon, have dedicated their entire lives to speaking on behalf of animals. There are thousands of yoga students all over the world who are vegan because of them. Guruji always said how pleased he was that Jivamukti was teaching *ahimsa* and vegetarianism. David and Sharon also founded Animal Mukti, a free spay-and-neuter clinic in New York City, with Janet Reinstra. They are a shining example of how to live harmoniously with the earth and all beings.

All the good flowing out of yoga centers encourages us to care. We want to care, but sometimes we forget, and so all of these places are reminding us: *Remember?*

The goodness in the world conducts itself through these individual people and their communities. Goodness uses the people who are willing to be instruments of goodness. They live and they work in collaboration. There's nothing egoistic about these individuals. It's goodness, and goodness is eternal. It never dies.

Getting Yelled At

Pointing out and correcting the drawbacks of Her children, the Holy Mother would say, "I am like a gardener. The garden is full of colorful flowers. I was not asked to look after the beautiful flowers, which are in no way defective. But I have been asked to remove the insects and worms from the pest-ridden flowers and plants. To remove the insects, I might have to pinch the petals and leaves, which is painful, but it is only to save the plants and flowers from destruction." In the same way, mother will always work with the children's weaknesses, the process of elimination is painful, but it is for your good. The virtuous aspects need no attention, but if your weaknesses are not removed, they will destroy your virtues as well. "My children, you may think that mother is angry with you, not at all. Mother loves you more than anyone else. And that is why she does all these things."

—A READING FROM AMMACHI, *A BIOGRAPHY OF MATA AMRITANANDAMAYI MA*

All my teachers have yelled at me, often. Guruji yelled at me so much that I developed a reputation for being yelled at by him. I loved having this reputation, and I loved being yelled at by him. It was what I missed most when I returned to India in the summer after he died.

Most people would agree that life seems overwhelming. We have to make decisions all the time, hoping those choices will be right, and wondering whether we have the tools to create the life we want. Life is coming at us and may make us feel confused and anxious and a little bit worried about everything all the time. Guruji thought his students were like that, worried all the time. Even in our better moments, that worry would still be there.

If you are a little worried all the time, and then the teacher yells at you, fiercely enough to nail your attention but with the love of a mother, the yelling cuts through the worry and lifts you out of it. It gives you the feeling that someone whom you esteem is going to guide you, show you, teach you, actually give you instructions, and it comes as a great relief. That's the experience of being yelled at by the great and holy teacher.

Then there's the memory of the experience, which creates a bond between yourself and the teacher. The bond lives inside you and enables you to go beyond any physical form. This enables you to go through life with less worry.

Like many great teachers, Ammachi travels often. Before Guruji took *mahasamadhi*, he traveled often. David Life and Sharon Gannon travel the globe, teaching. So we can't always be with the ones who yell at us. Built into the teacher–student relationship is the absence of the teachers. This gives us the blessed opportunity to miss them. The memory of being with them can be even clearer than the actual experience; the memory holds the sentiment. Yoga is a spiritual practice. In that way, the memory holds more power than the physical or material form. The memory is inside.

On September 11, 2001, when the two towers of the World Trade Center came down, Guruji was in New York City. He was teaching for the entire month of September. On the twelfth and thirteenth, classes were cancelled because no one was allowed to go to that part of the city. On the fourteenth, several hundred students came to the yoga class. Guruji didn't yell at anyone; he was unusually quiet. But, at the age of eighty-five, he got around and touched everyone, gently hit them on the head, tugged their arm, or tapped them on the rear end. I'm sure that for those people on that day, that touch from such a perfect man, while it lasted only a few seconds, left a memory that built a bond—a memory filled with a sentiment that would enable them to remold and shape themselves into the spiritual beings they yearned to be.

The Man with the Shaved Head, in the Vegetable Section

यद्यद् आचरति श्रेष्ठस् तत्तद् एवेतरो जनः ।
स यत् प्रमाणं कुरुते लोकस्तदनुवर्तते ॥ २१ ॥

yadyad ācarati śreṣṭhas tattad evetaro janaḥ
sa yat pramāṇaṃ kurute lokastadanuvartate

A great person leads by example, setting standards that are followed by others all over the world.

—*THE BHAGAVAD GITA*, CHAPTER THREE, VERSE 21

I was once in a health food store near where I live. I'd been busy and I hadn't bought any groceries in a while, and my husband was saying, "There's nothing to eat around here." The store in my neighborhood has organic produce and plenty of vegan cakes. It's clean and pleasant, and I was having a nice time in the vegetable section. A man who appeared to be Asian, had a shaved head, and was dressed like a monk caught my eye and I thought he looked nice. He smiled at me and I smiled back.

Then I looked in his cart—not deliberately, my eye just strayed in that direction. I saw that he had a head of broccoli, a beet, an onion, a couple of tomatoes and carrots, an orange, and a lemon. He had about eight different vegetables and a couple of tiny brown rolls. Everything in the cart was loose. Nothing was in a plastic bag; everything was there on its own. He had in his cart, too, a worn-out, empty canvas bag into which I assumed he would be putting his groceries.

Then my eyes focused on my cart, and what I had chosen was actually very similar to what he had: a head of broccoli, tomatoes, some collard greens, a couple of carrots, an onion, an orange, and a lime. But I had put each item into a plastic bag. I had nine plastic bags, a brown bag for my rolls, and no canvas bag.

One of the results of a yoga practice is that your vision changes, and when you look at anything, you're able to see the whole picture—the past, the present, and the future. You're able to see where things have come from and where things are going. Being a yogi for so many years, I'm beginning to use that skill. So when I looked inside that man's cart, I saw someone who cares about the world we live in. Here was someone who wasn't careless, but careful. He knew that those plastic bags that you pull and tear are not biodegradable. When they are disposed of, if they are dumped down on the ground, the earth becomes sick. If they are burned, the sky reddens and blackens and becomes sick. If the earth and the sky are sick, then the people will become sick, too. I looked into my cart and thought: "What carelessness, such waste and disregard!"

We don't need to ask ourselves what it would be like if the earth and the sky were sick, because we already know: it is happening. You might think, "What difference do nine plastic bags and a couple of brown bags make?" But, because of the law of karma, any action that you do is planting a seed for the next action, and you will do it a billion times over, into other lifetimes. So if we are careless, it will be a perpetual cycle. This other man, who was being thrifty, careful, and not wasteful, would do that over and over again.

I asked myself, "Where did I learn this? Using all these 'disposable bags'?" I was acting just like everybody else. I was, in essence, hypnotized, conditioned, mechanical, and that wasn't going to lead to enlightenment or to happiness. The other man wasn't acting just like everybody else. He was setting a good example.

People can *tell* you things. I mean, I know about the trees, and how they are being chopped down so fast to make products such as paper towels, paper cups, paper plates, paper bags, and . . . paper. I know how trees inhale carbon dioxide and exhale oxygen, and put moisture into the air, which is the seed for rain that nourishes the earth, purifies the air, and cools things down. The loss of that forest cover is one reason why we have global warming today. I know these things, but sometimes things go in one ear and out the other.

But when someone sets an example, like that lovely monk-like man, it is worth more than all the words in the world. That is why Krishna says, "Set a good example, the world will follow."

Teacher's Training

What needs doing, do it. Don't resist. Your balance must be dynamic, based on doing just the right thing, from moment to moment. Don't be a child, unwilling to grow up. Stereotyped gestures and postures will not help you. Rely entirely (not partially) on your clarity of thought, purity of motive, and integrity of action. Rely entirely on integrity of action. You cannot go wrong. You cannot go wrong.

—SHRI NISARGADATTA MAHARAJ, *I AM THAT*

This is the essential teaching of yoga. Integrity is the key to the door of God. If eighty percent of the time you have integrity, and twenty percent you don't, that twenty percent will imprison you. You have to rely entirely on your integrity. If you follow the instructions of your teachers well, than your actions will have integrity.

Sometimes I find myself in a situation where I feel stressed: s-t-r-e-s-s-e-d, *stressed.* Often the cause is that I have something important to do and don't feel I have enough time to do what I want to do well. Sometimes what happens if I'm in that state where I feel overwhelmed by that stress because I'm trying to do something quickly, somebody might come to me wanting something, and the tone of my voice might be gruff.

One morning, I had a great deal to do and I slept late. There was a knock on my door; someone was knocking at the door of a yogi. Think of those ancient stories! I'm sitting there among all of my sacred books, and I hear that knock. "Who is it?" I said with impatience in my most ferocious voice. It sounded almost frightening. I think I intimidated the person on the other side of the door. There was no response.

We do this when we feel stressed. We speak with a harsh tone to our fellow beings, and in justifying such behavior, grant ourselves the license to do so. The teachings say that one's integrity is to be fully present in basic human behaviors: for instance, in how I answer my door. That is the teaching that I have heard over and over. It's not only about rituals and *pujas*. It's about basic, decent behavior.

In 2005, I attended the Jivamukti Teacher Training graduation, as a student of mine was graduating. Her friend, who had graduated a year before, came to be supportive and brought with her a dozen long-stemmed white roses, each individually tied with a small bow. This way, the new graduate would have flowers to offer her teachers, mentors, roommates, and new friends.

The friend didn't bring the flowers so she could give them away; she brought them so someone else could give them away. That's intelligence, that's clarity of thought. The graduate had been studying and practicing intensely and wouldn't have had time to buy long-stemmed roses, but would want still to make offerings. The friend thought, "I'll provide the offerings. I'll do everything that needs to be done, but she can bring it to fruition." This is called giving your good karma away, and it's a very sacred teaching that our teachers have given us.

Sometimes, after a retreat or a journey to a distant land, we return feeling awakened, with a broader perspective, and a different outlook on things. Acts of integrity give us that sense of balance. After we have completed an act of integrity, we are awakened. It's as if we had gone on a great trip and met all the masters and received all the great teachings, and now we feel refreshed. If we incorporate integrity into our lives, it strengthens the bond that we have established with our teacher. There is a saying about the teacher–student bond, "The hand is in the glove and the fit is good."

Not Eating Meat

कट्वाम्लतीक्ष्णलवणोष्णहरीतशाक
सौवीरतैलतिलसर्षपमद्यमत्स्यान् ।
आजादिमांसदधितक्रकुलत्थकोल
पिण्याकहिङ्गुलशुनाद्यमपथ्यमाहुः ॥ ५९ ॥

kaṭvāmlatīkśṇalavaṇoṣṇaharītaśāka
sauvīratailatilasarṣapamadyamatsyān
ājādimāṃsadadhitakrakulatthakola
piṇyākahiṅgulaśunādyamapathyamāhuḥ

Bitter, sour, saltish, hot, green vegetables, fermented, oily, mixed with til seed, rape seed, intoxicating liquors, fish, meat, curds, horse gram, plums, oil cake, asafetida, garlic, onion, etc. should not be eaten.

—*THE HATHA YOGA PRADIPIKA*, CHAPTER ONE, VERSE 59

In November 2008, when my father passed away, my mother followed guidelines set down by the Jewish tradition of what to do when someone in the immediate family dies. For thirty days, my mother did things differently than she normally would. She didn't listen to music, watch television, or read a newspaper or novels. She didn't go out, handle money, or speak of anything other than my father. Many visitors of the community are supposed to come with provisions to enable a mourner to stay at home. The mourner is not supposed to eat meat at the meal immediately after the funeral. My mother did not eat meat for the full thirty days.

My mother was happy to follow those rules. It felt strange for me to be in the house without any classical music playing, without my mom doing the crossword puzzle in the *New York Times*, or without her going out.

Several months later, I returned to visit her, and her life was mostly back to normal. But one of the things I noticed after having been with her for a few days was that she wasn't eating any meat. She's always liked meat, and we've argued about this for over thirty years.

"You haven't gone back to eating meat," I said.

"Yes," she replied.

"How was it for those thirty days?" I asked.

"Actually, it wasn't difficult at all," she said. "It felt natural."

"Oh, why is that?"

"Well, I was beside myself with unhappiness," she responded. "I had reached a point of such extreme suffering that I just couldn't cause any more suffering. I did not want to eat animals."

I think sometimes it takes extreme pain to sober us up so that we can understand what we're doing and why from a new viewpoint. If we look truthfully at what we're doing and find in any place in our lives compassion that we've repressed, then that repressed compassion will be counter-productive to any kind of healing process. In order to feel human in some kind of totality, repressed compassion needs to be transformed to allow the mercy that we naturally have as human beings to flow.

En Theos

उत्साहात्साहसाद्धैर्यात्तत्त्वज्ञानाश्च निश्चयात् ।
जनसङ्गपरित्यागात्षड्भिर्योगः प्रसिद्ध्यति ॥ १६ ॥

utsāhāt sāhasāddhairyāt tattva jnānāś ca niścayāt
janasanga parityāgāt ṣaḍbhir yogaḥ prasiddhyati

The following six bring speedy success: courage, daring, perseverance, discriminative knowledge, faith, aloofness from company.

—*THE HATHA YOGA PRADIPIKA*, CHAPTER ONE, VERSE 16

This verse is found at the beginning of *The Hatha Yoga Pradipika*, and it lists certain qualities that are necessary for succeeding in yoga. Without them, the practices themselves won't work. Before any of the instructions are given—how to fast, how to use enemas, how to drink ten glasses of salt water, how to look at the tip of your nose, how to brush your skin rapidly, how to do *pacchimotonasana* (the seated forward bend), or how to breathe correctly—we are reminded of what our attitude should be. Great importance is attached to acting with the right kind of behavior.

The first quality that's listed in this verse is enthusiasm. We cannot succeed in yoga if we lack enthusiasm. Scripture is intended to be read and contemplated. Thus, it's good to ponder, "What is enthusiasm?"

My husband Robert and I went to the Berkshires in western Massachusetts for his birthday. A community of Sufis lives there, and we wanted to visit. I was mentioning this to one of my students, and she said, "I have a house in that area, why don't you stay there?"

"That won't be necessary," I replied, "we can stay with the Sufis."

"We won't be there," my student said, "but I would love it so much if you stayed there. Why don't I give you the key just in case you decide you'd like to stay there?"

"Okay," I responded, and took the keys. I think I may even still have them.

On our way to the Sufis, we decided to swing by my student's house to see what it looked like. It was beautiful, down a winding dirt road, far from traffic and noise, and deep inside nature. It stood on a hill and it presented bucolic views. It contained many rooms. We discovered that the owners, my friend and her husband, collect art, and we came upon many paintings and old photographs throughout the house.

We slept in an antique wooden bed built in Bali, with carvings of flowers and animals. We had to step into this bed. I'd never slept in anything like it. It must have been intended for a queen from a dynasty far away and perhaps long gone. My student—our absent hostess—had an extensive library, and one night we sat up late, pulling out all the books.

After we had been there for a few days, I thought I'd better call her because I had indicated that we probably wouldn't stay at her house, and now we had been there already for three days, having a great time. I called her and she said, "Oh, are you at my house?"

"Yes, I'm using your phone."

I heard her shouting to her husband, "They're at the house! They're at the house!" She was so enthusiastic, to offer her home to her yoga teacher.

I received a gas bill that was unusually high. I knew it couldn't be right, so I called the gas company and spoke with someone who said he would come over to read the meter. There's no buzzer to get into the building, so when this fellow arrived, he would need to call me from a cell phone.

"Do you have a cell phone?" I asked the man.

"No," he replied, "but I have to get one because my wife is ill and needs to be able to reach me."

I didn't know this man personally; he was simply the individual at the gas company to whom I was expressing my aggravation about my bill. That night, however, when I was saying my prayers, I began to pray for that man and his wife, and all the people who need cell phones because a loved one is sick or possibly in danger. I still think about that man and his wife often.

I'm enthusiastic about the fact that I prayed. I'm enthusiastic because his statement didn't just flit by me but stayed with me. I'm enthusiastic that the concern I have for others is growing. Enthusiasm for the positive qualities one has helps those qualities to grow. Enthusiasm for the spiritual teachings motivates us to put them into practice. Enthusiasm about one's birth as a human helps one not to waste it. My student was enthusiastic that she had a home she could offer to others. We have to be enthusiastic if we are going to experience yoga. Enthusiasm comes from the Greek en *theos,* which means in *God.*

A Blade of Grass

आत्मौपम्येन सर्वत्र समं पश्यति योऽर्जुन ।
सुखं वा यदि वा दुःखं स योगी परमो मतः ॥ ३२ ॥

ātmaupamyena sarvatra samaṃ paśyati yo'rjuna
sukhaṃ vā yadi vā dukḥaṃ sa yogī paramo mataḥ

He is a perfect yogi who, by comparison to his own self, sees the true equality of all beings, in both their happiness and their distress, O Arjuna!

—*THE BHAGAVAD GITA*, CHAPTER SIX, VERSE 32

The great American poet Walt Whitman (1819–1892) wrote a long poem that had to do with the soul and called it "Song of Myself." In the poem is a passage where a young boy and a man are together in a field of grass. The child plucks some grass, holds it in his "full hands," shows the man, and asks, "What is the grass?" The old man wonders how to answer the boy's question. "How could I answer the child?" he writes. "I do not know what it is any more than he." But the man feels that he must answer the child:

> I guess it must be the flag of my disposition, out of hopeful green stuff woven.
>
> Or I guess it is the handkerchief of the Lord,
> A scented gift and remembrancer designedly dropped,

Bearing the owner's name someway in the corners, that we may see and remark, and say Whose?

Or I guess the grass is itself a child . . . the produced babe of the vegetation.

Then he adds that the grass is the same that grows among different peoples—"among black folks as among white, / Kanuck, Tuckahoe, Congressman, Cuff"—and he concludes with the insight that the grass now seems to him "the beautiful uncut hair of graves."(1) It is my reading of this passage that the narrator has proved to the little boy that there is no such thing as death.

During the Civil War, Whitman, who had been living in the city of Brooklyn, decided to stop writing poetry and volunteered as a nurse in a hospital in Washington D.C., where there were many wounded soldiers. He learned how to clean and bandage wounds, and grew close to the soldiers. They told him about their lives, their stories, their feelings, and he was moved. Because he was a great poet, it came about that the soldiers asked, "Would you write a letter for my mother? My son? My wife? I want to tell them how much I miss them. Could you make it poetic? Could you tell my wife I think she is beautiful? Could you compare her to the grass?"

Whitman wrote hundreds of letters while he was cleaning these wounds. He later said that this period in his life, so full of sadness, was also the most joyful because he connected with these soldiers. That is what joy is. Joy is empathy. That is why when we see His Holiness the Dalai Lama, who has seen extreme suffering and experienced great hardship, he is often laughing and smiling because of his empathy.

(1) Quoted from Walt Whitman, *The Complete Poems*, edited with an introduction by Francis Murphy (New York: Penguin Books, 2004). The ellipsis is in the original.

Precious Books

ते ह्लादपरितापफलाः पुण्यापुण्यहेतुत्वात् ॥ १४ ॥

te hlāda paritāpa phalāḥ puṇyāpuṇya hetutvāt

The karmas bear fruits of pleasure and pain caused by merit and demerit.

—MASTER PATANJALI'S *YOGA SUTRAS*, BOOK TWO, SUTRA 14

A long time ago, some people who weren't yet enlightened and whose minds were not completely pure read the Hebrew Scriptures and came across a verse that says, "An eye for an eye, a tooth for a tooth." It is a phrase that occurs in various forms in the books of Exodus, Leviticus, and Deuteronomy, although it initially appeared in the code of laws developed by Hammurabi, who ruled Babylon in Mesopotamia nearly four thousand years ago. So it is obviously a very ancient sentiment.

At their ordinary level of understanding, these readers of the Scriptures interpreted the phrase to mean that if someone plucks another's eye out, it's all right to pluck that individual's out in turn. They disseminated that interpretation in the way that gossip spreads, not really understanding what they were talking about. These people then said that revenge was good, because it says so in the Bible, and they used that argument to back up any kind of vengefulness that they partook of. There were others, equally unenlightened, who took in this verse and said, "This is bad. Revenge is bad. So the Bible is a bad book."

I have heard this often, that the Bible is a book about revenge. This assumption seeps into the consciousness of people who become infected with these low-level interpretations or misconceptions that are spread around. These ideas last over centuries, so that even people who have never read these scriptures believe what they've heard.

After the two planes crashed into the World Trade Center in lower Manhattan on the morning of September 11, 2001, the media implied that all the people who shared the religion of those believed to be behind these acts of extreme violence were to be feared. This kind of talk goes on all the time. Everywhere, people argue about whose book is the word of God, whose religion is the best, and what nations are evil. They say this and they say that. Ignorance increases, and it becomes very hard to free oneself of this conditioning.

The sutra from Master Patanjali's *Yoga Sutras* states that a good deed bears good fruit and a bad deed produces bad fruit. If our conversations are divisive and we talk about things that we don't properly understand, then the world around us will reflect back this turmoil. The world is an echo. The Indians make it very simple. They say, "If you plant an apple seed, you get an apple tree. If you want a peach tree, don't plant an apple seed." In different words, we would say "An eye for an eye and a tooth for a tooth." But this law of karma doesn't give us license to pluck out another person's eye and find that all right. It means rather: As ye reap so shall you sow. To use sacred books to support any kind of violence is to misuse them.

Through contemplation and love, one begins to see that all sacred books carry the same message: unity. One sees past whose book it is and who wrote it—past the appearance, past the words, to the truth: God is one.

A Quality of Readiness

Venerable Thupten Jinpa, a Tibetan Buddhist monk, has lived in the United States for many years and was born and raised in Haiti. After the earthquake in January 2010, the monk lost contact with his father, and wanted to go to Haiti to look for him. Considering the situation, he thought it best not to go alone—he hoped for an assistant, perhaps one with health-care skills. So he asked his lama, Geshe Michael Roach, if he knew of someone, and Geshela said he would put out an e-mail to his *sanga* (community), which totals over a thousand people, and certainly someone would respond. My best friend, Lisa Schrempp, who is an Ayurvedic doctor and a long-time yoga practitioner, responded.

When Venerable Jinpa received Lisa's call, he said he was surprised. Somehow he was expecting a man to call. But he agreed to meet her anyway. At the end of the meeting, he told her he appreciated her concern, but that he thought she might be too fragile for the task and that he would continue to look for someone else. She wished him all the best and that was that.

A week passed and no one else from the *sanga* called the monk. So he called Lisa saying that, if she was still willing to go, he was leaving in two days. She told him that she was still willing and ready to leave. And so, two days later, she left for Port-au-Prince with two large suitcases full of supplies.

Why was Lisa the only one who responded to the e-mail? It is because she was ready. She has a quality of readiness. The masters always say, "Are you ready?" Ready for what, really? Ready to see the suffering of mankind. Ready to see God in the intensity of life. Lisa was ready. Where does that readiness come from? All the challenges that she has faced and not escaped have made her ready. In the same way, this new challenge will make her ready for something else that is contained in her future.

There is something known and something unknown. Lisa knows she is ready. Even the monk stating he would look for someone else didn't plant any doubts in her mind. She knew she had the continuing blessing of her gurus, lamas, and teachers, and she knew what that was worth. She knew that if she was going to Haiti, it would be good for her to be with a monk. These are things she knew. This is real knowledge.

When she made her decision, Lisa didn't know what she would find in Port-au-Prince, what it would be like to be in a city that had endured such destruction, where there was already so much poverty. She didn't know how it would unfold for her. But what she *did* know made her ready to step into the unknown, and it is there that we feel a greatness of life and we grow.

In the famous novella *A Christmas Carol* by Charles Dickens, the ghost of Christmas present wearing a cape appears before the miser Scrooge. Scrooge asks to see what's inside the cape, since it is bulging slightly, and when the spirit opens its cape, Scrooge is faced with two starving children, who represent Ignorance and Want. It is this moment that helps to prepare Scrooge to change his way of life.

✲ ✲ ✲

What Lisa found in Port-au-Prince was a city of sadness and trauma, rubble and darkness. Though it was raining, most people and even the dogs preferred to stay outdoors, afraid that the remaining structures would continue to collapse. Most businesses were closed, but people were selling food on the roadside. Many were cold and hungry, some were lost.

At the same time, Lisa found a quality of reassurance, because so many people came from all over to be of help. Lisa's hands-on treatments (mostly in the context of Ayurvedic massage) were given without proper time or supplies, but she felt they were effective, especially among the children. One day, she gave almost two hundred children treatments. Lisa said that when people realized that she had come to help, they welcomed the assistance, and accepted it without resistance or cynicism. She said most people didn't have it in them to say *thank you* after the treatments, but they would walk away slightly more hopeful.

When we embrace the suffering of others, we get something back. My friend will get something back for going to Haiti to help in a city of almost two million people after a terrible earthquake, and what she receives she will feel grateful for. But something may not come right away. First, she may have had to be content with the suffering. We must not expect an instant return. But eventually, we get back equal to what we give.

The Guru's Breath Count

यमनियमासनप्राणायामप्रत्याहारधारणाध्यानसमाधयोऽष्टावाङ्गानि ॥ २९ ॥

yamaniyamāsanaprāṇāyāmapratyāhāra
dhāraṇādhyānasamādhayo'ṣṭāvāṅgani

Restraint, observance, posture, breath control, sense withdrawal, concentration, meditation, and absorption are the eight limbs of yoga.

—MASTER PATANJALI'S *YOGA SUTRAS*,
BOOK TWO, SUTRA 29

Guruji taught Ashtanga yoga: *yama niyama asana pranayama pratyahara dharana dhyana Samadhi.* The way he taught *asana* was in series—one, two, three, etc. We thought the series were fixed. On Fridays, Guruji would lead primary series. After years of calling it a certain way, he would take us by surprise and change something. His change usually meant adding something especially hard, and lengthening the breath count. We would do things that way for a while, until we thought it was fixed, and then he would surprise us and change it, making it more difficult, with longer breath counts. Over the two decades that I had the great fortune of being in some of those led classes, they changed and they got harder, never easier. The hardest of these classes took place shortly before Guruji died. He had stopped teaching completely, but came downstairs and taught one class anyway.

We have all these fixed notions about ourselves and about others. Breaking down our fixed notions is the guru's undertaking, while encouraging us to accept change, impermanence, and difficulty. The challenges in Guruji's yoga class totally exhausted our acquired strength. This is how we found our innate strength. Our innate strength is our real strength, but we'll never find it if we don't work hard. This is why whenever Guruji made things harder, he'd say, "Now, easy!"

The Jackfruit Tree

आत्मौपम्येन सर्वत्र समं पश्यति योऽर्जुन ।
सुखं वा यदि वा दुःखं स योगी परमो मतः ॥ ३२ ॥

ātmaupamyena sarvatra samaṃ paśyati yo'rjuna
sukhaṃ vā yadi vā dukḥaṃ sa yogī paramo mataḥ

O Arjuna, the best type of yogi is he who feels for others whether in grief or pleasure, even as he feels for himself.

—*THE BHAGAVAD GITA,* CHAPTER SIX, VERSE 32

Dr. Gurudat, my music teacher in India, used to live in a very nice house in Mysore, the most beautiful town in the world. His house stood in an area that is serene, quiet, pleasant, shady, and cool even on hot days, because of the many trees. The house was spacious, and there was one room off to the side, just for music lessons. At the back of the house was the kitchen, and through the kitchen door, was their back yard. In the back yard a beautiful jackfruit tree grew. The fruit tastes like a sweet avocado. There was a hibiscus bush, too, with large pink flowers. Dr. Gurudat's wife, Chandrika, would make vegetarian stews from the jackfruit and would pick flowers off the bush every day and bring them inside and decorate the pictures of the gurus, gods, and ancestors with them.

Inevitably, each year that I studied with Dr. Gurudat, Chandrika would make a meal for me. Somehow, she always knew what my favorite dishes were. She's a traditional Indian woman, quiet and reserved, who never spoke much to me, but somehow in the meals that she prepared I felt that she expressed to me a very positive quality about life.

Then, a few years ago, Dr. Gurudat had to leave his position of teaching law and look elsewhere for work. He seemed dispirited. Finally, he found work three hours from Mysore, in Bangalore, a city that is polluted and densely populated, with much more poverty and crime. So the family moved there and rented an apartment in a building, with people living on top of them and underneath them.

When I went to visit them in Bangalore, Chandrika made a meal for me. I sat and ate the meal and it was tasteless. At the end of the meal, I felt that Chandrika had, as in Mysore, without talking to me, expressed herself through her meal. I felt that what she had expressed was not the positive quality about life that I had felt before, but rather how much she was missing her jackfruit tree and her hibiscus bush. Her sadness was hidden in the food. When I left, I hugged her and said, "I hope you can return to Mysore soon."

Now when I say my prayers, Chandrika appears and a special feeling comes over me. Those moments I feel for her linger. Mostly we pray for and think about ourselves first, and that's because our tendency (*samskara*) to put ourselves first is so deep-rooted. So we go, around and around the wheel of *samskara*, thinking mostly about ourselves.

Sometimes, it may be appropriate to pray for oneself, but our prayers should not be limited to ourselves, or they will create more separation. This past April 2010, a terrible explosion took place in the middle of the Gulf of Mexico, causing oil to gush into the ocean. More than a month later, the oil was still gushing out of control and the clean up was slow. I wanted to go there and see the birds and the fish dead and dying. Somehow it was not enough just to know about it. So I prayed for them. Our prayers should take us back to our connection to others.

Brush with Death

उत्तानं शववद्भूमौ शयनं तच्छवासनम् ।
शवासनं श्रान्तिहरं चित्तविश्रान्तिकारकम् ॥ ३४ ॥

uttānaṃ śavavadbhūmau śayanaṃ tacchavāsanam
śavāsanaṃ śrāntiharaṃ cittaviśrānti kārakam

Lying flat on the ground with the face upwards like a corpse is savasana.

—*THE HATHA YOGA PRADIPIKA*, CHAPTER ONE, VERSE 32

In the Bihar School of Yoga edition of *The Hatha Yoga Pradipika* there is a drawing of a man lying down with a caption underneath that reads "Like a corpse." Maharishi Swatmarama is instructing us to practice death.

Life is made up of moments, hours, days, weeks, months, years, and decades. Like that, we drift through life. For many people, drifting through life is a blur. Then, something occurs, such as a brush with death, and you awaken from that blur and see life as something more precious than before. You're almost leveled, and the experience makes you less harsh and more gentle.

The yogi doesn't want to wait for a brush with death, an experience that some people don't undergo until they actually die. *Savasana* is a practice that puts the practitioner in a space that's poignant, as when you are dying, where everything slows down and becomes distinct. You put yourself in that kind of space so that afterwards you see things with more clarity.

My husband's mother has lived in New York City for decades and has all of her favorite places she goes to for bread, flowers, soup, fabric, and bonbons. Now that she's in her late eighties, however, she can't trudge all over Manhattan to get what she wants, so she goes to the deli on the corner.

"I accept it," she said to me one day. "I can't walk to buy the specialty items. The deli is right there." Now that she was old and no longer out and about, working and busy, she added, she had to stay in. "You know what I do when I stay in?" she continued. "I go into myself and gather. I gather, and I have realizations, and I'm glad I've gotten old. Now, I have time to have realizations."

"What are your realizations?" I asked her.

"Well, I'm not telling," she responded. "They're *my* realizations. If I told one to you, it would make it less." Then she added, "Do you understand what I mean?"

"Yes," I said. "I understand what you mean."

"That's good," she said. "We get along well."

We need to have our own realizations, and we don't need to tell them. That's not what realizations are for. Realizations are for waking up. Practicing death, *savasana,* means lying down, not sleeping, not doing anything . . . except waking up. The specific placement of your body, horizontal and on the floor, as low as you can get and in an upside-down prostration, is not egoistic. No one boasts, "My *savasana* is really great!" in the way one might about a one-armed handstand. That humility is the death of the ego; that is what we're practicing in *savasana.*

Voices in Our Heads

ऋतं वदिष्यामि सत्यं वदिष्यामि तन्मामवतु तदवक्तारमवतु अवतुमाम अवतु वक्तारं ॐ शान्तिः शान्तिः शान्तिः

ṛtaṃ vadiṣyāmi satyaṃ vadiṣyāmi tanmāmavatu tadvaktāramavatu avatu mām avatu vaktāraṃ oṁ śāntiḥ śāntiḥ śāntiḥ

May I seek only the right. May I seek only the truth.
May that protect me. May that protect my teacher. May spiritual knowledge shine forth. AUM, peace, peace, peace.

—FROM *THE SHANTIH MANTRAS*, THE GREAT PRAYERS FOR PEACE

There is so much suffering in the world that we feel the need to put something good into the universe. These ancient mantras and songs are said to invoke peace.

Nadam is inner sound. The questions arise for the yogi, "What sounds are helpful to listen to? Does a mood of kindness affect how we listen? What voices do we hear in our head?" There are many different inner sounds. The enlightened ones talk about the celestial music they hear. We have that to look forward to.

One form of inner sound is the voice of our conscience. This is something that inhabits all of us, although some of us don't hear it as well as others. When we do a bad deed, a voice inside us says, "That was bad." Along with this voice, we feel a vibration and a disturbance. It may be hard to sleep or breathe, and we may feel that things are closing in on us.

Similarly, when we do a good deed, a voice inside says, "That was good." Along with that voice we experience a vibration, and we feel at ease, and we enjoy a sense that we are using our time well.

If we do a bad deed, without anyone punishing us from outside, inside we hear a punitive voice; if we do a good deed, without anyone rewarding us from outside, inside we hear the voice of reward. This is the voice of conscience, of the higher self, the true teacher, or *satguru,* and we must listen to it. For this reason, we have an *asana* practice, so that we can quiet down and hear.

The cashier in the store gives you ten dollars extra in change and the voice in you says, "Great! I'll get a soy cappuccino with this extra money." But another voice says, "That's wrong." So you can either keep the money or listen to the voice that's pointing out that you're stealing. People are gossiping, saying mean things about another human being, and a voice in you says, "This is entertaining. Join in!" But another voice says, "Run! Get out of this room quickly." You have a choice.

I was in my car, running late. I was facing the green light, but a man in front of me was slowly crossing the street. I was about to beep my horn when I thought, "Do I want to live like this? Do I really want to be out there just honking my horn? I mean, he's got to get to the other side. Just let him be."

Our conscience is said by some to be what makes us different from animals. But I'm sure animals hear that inner voice, too. When we hear the *satguru,* but then ignore it, we are in effect taking a stone and building a wall between ourselves and God. Eventually, we would become profoundly alienated, far away from the source of wisdom and bliss; yet we ourselves have built that wall.

It's crucial that when we hear that lower voice, that puny and selfish voice, we resolve not to listen to it any longer. If we don't listen to it, it inevitably goes away, and we become lovelier every moment of our lives.

Refraining from Speaking

ॐ पूर्णमदः पूर्णमिदं पूर्णात् पूर्णमुदच्यते ।
पूर्णस्य पूर्णमादाय पूर्णमेवावशिष्यते ॥
ॐ शान्तिः शान्तिः शान्तिः

oṃ pūrṇamadaḥ pūrṇamidaṃ pūrṇat pūrṇamudacyate
pūrṇasya pūrṇamādāya pūrṇamevavaśiṣyate
oṃ śāntiḥ śāntiḥ śāntiḥ

Purna is full, whole, intact, complete, perfect, golden, fat with goodness, fat with joy, robust. No matter what you give, what you're left with is full, and what you give is full. It is perfect, it is whole, it is complete, it is fat.

—AN INVOCATION FROM *THE ISHA UPANISHAD*

Purna means full, intact, complete, perfect—fat, actually. Teachers say that in order to experience that fullness or satisfaction or satiation, silence is helpful.

Once, when I was visiting my parents, my brother and father were having a conversation about physics, magnetics, lubrication, and spectroscopy. I was silent, because I didn't have a clue what they were talking about, so I had nothing to say. That is not the kind of silence that the spiritual masters are referring to. Rather, it is where one *could* say something but instead you choose to be silent.

On another occasion, I had received some wonderful news, felt greatly excited, and began to make long-distance phone calls to tell people of my news. I was speaking to a dear friend who was going through a difficult time. She was crying on the phone, and I thought, "This isn't a good time to share my news." It was a little hard for me to restrain myself, but I knew that she needed someone to listen to her, so I remained silent. I refrained from speaking and provided a good ear.

I was at the airport at five o'clock one morning, and came across men shouting at each other, using very crude language. I was ready to tell them a thing or two when my husband took my hand and started walking to a different section of the airport. Most often, when people are bothering you, it is better to refrain than to give them a piece of your mind.

An ashram in southern India where I like to go is called Ananda Ashram: it is Papa Ram Dass's place. They have eight cows there who are probably the best cared-for cows in the world. The residents of the ashram sing mantras to them and hang garlands of flowers around their necks. As a result, the milk and curd taste different. Unlike many of the cows in India, these cows are well fed on fresh grass.

I should say that the experience of cows at Ananda Ashram is *extremely* rare, not only in India but around the world. Approximately three-and-a-half million of our sister cows are slaughtered in the United States every day. Their bodies are used as machines, because of their reproductive capabilities. When they can no longer provide milk, they are taken to slaughter to become a "steak" or "burger." Their calves are stolen and skinned to make a pair of shoes or a purse. So the cows at Ananda are very fortunate.

Early in the morning at Ananda, an old man walks down the driveway and opens the main gate to the ashram to find a truckload of grass. In the middle of the night, someone leaves grass for the cows. Whoever it is has remained silent for the last twenty-five years and doesn't want any credit. At the ashram they say, "We do not know who is giving us this grass."

Anonymous giving is a wonderful form of silence. In moments of silence, the mind is serene, and in that wavelessness, something of the profound nature of life is experienced, and life is full.

The Antidote to Unhappiness

सर्वे भवन्तु सुखिनः सर्वे सन्तु निरामयाः
सर्वे भद्राणि पश्यन्तु मा कश्चित् दुःखभाग्भवेत्

sarve bhavantu sukhinaḥ sarve santu nirāmayāḥ
sarve bhadrāṇi paśyantu mā kaścit duḥkha bhāgbhavet

May all be happy. May all be free from sickness. May all see what is good and beautiful. May no one be unhappy.

—A TRADITIONAL PRAYER BEFORE CLASS

The spiritual person has many prayers to benefit others—mantras, where one expresses one's wish that others should be happy. But of course, the individual wants to be happy as well. This is hard because in some measure we are always unhappy; even in our happiest moments, there is some unhappiness. We sense that something is not quite right. This unhappiness is hard to get rid of because it is so deep-rooted and we're not sure where it comes from. It's abstract. Even if we thought we knew where it came from, we would not know how to reach in and fix it.

But being good and kind to others, trying to please them and make them happy, works as an antidote to our unhappiness. Making others happy makes us happy, too.

By far the happiest person I've known was my guru. Not only was he happy, but he made many people happy, and even said so.

But Guruji also had a lot of sadness in him. He was sad when his wife died; he was sad that tigers are going extinct in the wild, and that the forests in India are being cut down. He was sad when a yoga practitioner was not vegetarian. He was sad if he saw yoga students being unfriendly toward each other. He was sad if someone killed a mosquito. He was sad at the state of the world. He read the paper often and would cry. But his sadness never threatened or diminished his happiness. His happiness was so large that it had room for sadness.

I was very fortunate to spend almost twenty summers with Guruji. At the end of one summer, I said to him, "Guruji on Wednesday I'm leaving."

"Oh," Guruji said. "Why?" (He asked "Why?" a lot, and in his presence, it was difficult to remember why.)

When I went to say *goodbye,* Guruji looked at me: "You happy?"

"Oh yes, Guruji," I replied, "very happy."

"You happy?" he asked again.

"Yes, Guruji."

"Happy you?"

"Yes, yes, happy, happy."

"Happy happy?"

"Yes, yes."

Then he looked concerned. "You. . . ." He paused. "Keep it. . . . Keep it."

Guruji knew how hard it is to keep happiness. I would come home from India and after a while I would start losing my happiness, and then I would hear him yelling, "Keep it."

The happiness that we gain from our practices should not be squandered. It's fragile and we can wreck it with the wrong activities. But if we keep it, then it will build, and as it builds, it automatically spreads to others.

For Steven

तत्र प्रत्ययैक तानता ध्यानम् ॥ २ ॥

tatra pratyayaika tānatā dhyānam

Dhyana is the continuous flow, the unbroken stream of stretching in one direction toward the holy object.

—MASTER PATANJALI'S *YOGA SUTRAS*, BOOK THREE, SUTRA 2

I have a friend named Steven who moved from New York City to Florida to live with his parents because he was diagnosed with cancer and had become very sick. I decided to visit him. Even though he was unwell, he wanted to pick me up at the airport. I assured him that I was a world traveler and would be able to find my way, but he insisted. When he came to meet me, he arrived in his father's white convertible, with the top down. He had a cloth sack attached to his stomach in place of his colon. He suggested that, if I was not too tired, we could drive a little out of the way to an island with many exotic plants.

"Sure," I said.

So we drove to the island and Steven showed me flowering bushes that he told me were a hundred years old. He pointed out that the same blossoms came in different colors.

"Look, Lady Ruth!" he said. "This is the same flower in yellow, in purple, in blue, and in white."

He asked me to smell the ones he knew were particularly fragrant. He knew how much I love flowers. It made him happy to take me to see them.

Birds and butterflies were everywhere. Steven called the butterflies "flying flowers" after a poem by Guy de Maupassant. I was touched that, even as he was dying, Steven appreciated the beauty of a flower or simply its fragrance. In Sanskrit, there is a word, *tanata*: Master Patanjali uses it in the *Yoga Sutras* to describe meditation. It means to stretch. In yoga class we stretch in many ways—we even stretch our breath. *Tanata* refers mostly to stretching one's mind: stretching one's mind to the holiness of an object like the beauty of a flower.

Later, in the car, Steven told me that since he'd become sick, everyone had been kind to him: close friends, strangers, and even the people whom he had previously not gotten along with. He said that through his illness he had learned that deep down everyone is good. Sometimes this can feel like a stretch. But this is what yoga teaches. This is the optimistic message of yoga: that human beings are innately good. We don't have to go out and obtain goodness. We just have to stretch ourselves toward it. It is already inside us; it is to be uncovered, not manufactured. We have an unlimited supply.

Life's Interruptions

त्रयम् एकत्र संयमः ॥ ४ ॥

trayam ekatra saṃyamaḥ

The practice of dharana, dhyana, and Samadhi upon one object is called samyama.

—MASTER PATANJALI'S *YOGA SUTRAS*, BOOK THREE, SUTRA 4

Enlightenment, for a wave in the ocean, is the moment the wave realizes it is water.

—THICH NHAT HANH

The simultaneous practice of *dharana* (concentration with interruptions), *dhyana* (concentration without interruptions, also called meditation), and *Samadhi* (absorption with the object of concentration) is called *samyama*. *Tryam* is three, *eka* is one. Turning the three into one is *samyama*. As Master Patanjali says, these three things exist simultaneously, *ekatra*—in one place.

When I was a little girl, my mother would put me in my bed and say, "I'm going downstairs to paint, while you go to sleep."

I'd say, "Okay. I'll try to go to sleep."

My mother would put on a multicolored floral smock and go down to the basement, where she kept an easel. She'd put on classical music and turn the volume up quite high considering that I was supposed to be sleeping, and she'd paint. After a little while, I'd tiptoe out of my room, sit at the top of the stairs, and peek down at my mom. I'd be quiet, but after a while I'd want her attention.

So I'd continue downstairs and say, "Mom, I'm having trouble sleeping."

"I told you not to interrupt me," she would say. "I'm painting. Now, go back upstairs."

"But can't you just tell me a story?" I'd ask.

"I'm painting and don't wish to be interrupted," she'd insist. "Go back upstairs."

"But Mom," I'd whine. "Can't you just tell me *one* story?"

"Ruth, I'm fresh out of stories. I don't have any stories for you that I can tell."

"I'm sure there must be one story that you could tell me."

"Well, did I ever tell you the story about my hunchback cousin?"

"No," I'd say, "you never told me that one."

"No?" My mother would act surprised. "I didn't tell you? He has an estate in England. Let's go upstairs and I'll tell you the story."

Just like that, my mother would interrupt her painting and classical music, take off her smock to come upstairs, and tell me the story. It was always great. She's a great storyteller.

In this passage, I think Master Patanjali is telling us not to flip out when our meditation is interrupted. *Samyama* is interrupted concentration, uninterrupted concentration, and absorption. It's all happening at the same time. The interruptions in meditation are part of the meditation. We can continue and nothing is ruined.

The interruptions in life are life.

One By One

Guruji didn't speak much English and had a few expressions that he used over and over again. One of them that he seemed really to enjoy using was, "One by one. Yes, one by one."

It used to be that Guruji taught in a room with enough space for only twelve students. Those who were waiting to get in would sit on the stairs directly outside of the classroom. When someone would finish the practice and a space would open, Guruji would call in the next student. "Yes, one by one, one by one you come. Yes, one by one." And he seemed really to love saying this.

One year, I had injured my left hamstring, and I could feel the pain and the strain in every pose. A year later, it was better, and then I pulled my right hamstring. When I told Guruji that now I had injured my right hamstring, his reply was familiar.

"Yes, one by one. One by one," he said. "Overhauling. Overhauling. No problem. One by one."

There are 84,000 *asanas*, and when I was younger I wanted to attempt all of them. Guruji advised against it. "No, no. One by one," he said. Once, I had to wait five years before I was granted the next posture. I have thought about that often over the years. "One by one. One by one."

If you think of a bird building a nest, the bird goes and finds a twig and brings it back, and goes and fetches another twig and brings it back. Then he finds a piece of string and brings it back and finds another twig and brings it back. One by one, he builds a nest.

This was what Guruji was teaching us. Doing something step-by-step amounts to transformation. There's a saying, "Pade, pade," which means foot by foot, or "One by one."

* * *

The Jivamuktea Café offers a dish called "Choice of Three." Suppose you order spirulina millet, black beans, and kale. First, you eat the millet, then the kale, and then the beans. When you're finished with the last spoonful of beans, you're full. But it's not just the last spoonful of beans that makes you full. It's everything that came before it. *Sadhana,* or spiritual work, is said to be like that; every step along the way is crucial.

My Father's Light

विशोका वा ज्योतिष्मती ॥ ३६ ॥

viśōkā vā jyotiṣmatī

Visoka is sorrowlessness and jyotish is brightness.

—MASTER PATANJALI'S *YOGA SUTRAS*, BOOK ONE, SUTRA 36

In November 2008, my father, Lothar Lauer, died. Two weeks later I was in New York City, where Geshe Michael Roach and Lama Christie were giving two weeks of classes on *The Hatha Yoga Pradipika.* I missed most of the classes because I had been in California for my dad's funeral. When I returned, I wanted to attend the remaining classes.

On Wednesday, Geshela requested, "Lady Ruth, will you sing Book Four of *The Hatha Yoga Pradipika* at the class on Friday?"

I hesitated. "Geshela, I really don't feel up for it right now; my father just passed away." But Geshela said a few things (he was extraordinarily persuasive) and twisted my arm. I couldn't say no to him.

The night I was scheduled to sing, I was already outside of my apartment about to go to the class, when I turned around and went back in. I have a picture of my dad in a large frame that was taken shortly before he died. I grabbed it, wrapped it in a towel, and put it in my bag. I wasn't sure why I was bringing it, but I did so nonetheless.

I arrived at the event, and when it was time for me to sing, the Lamas lifted me from the floor onto a little stage. On the stage rested many pictures of the Buddha, piles of flower petals and bouquets, and deep red cushions on which the Lamas had been sitting for the past two weeks.

I slid the picture of my father out of my bag and leaned it against a vase of flowers.

Geshela turned and said, "Oh, is that your father?"

"Yes," I replied.

"He looks like Geshe Lothar," he responded. Geshe Lothar is one of Geshela's heart Lamas. I was happy that the photo of my father reminded him of his teacher.

Then we sang: one Jimi Hendrix song, all of Chapter Four of *The Hatha Yoga Pradipika,* and a few of my favorite verses from *The Bhagavad Gita.* It was an hour of singing and it was two o'clock in the morning when we were done. Several hundred people were gathered, and when we finished, an indescribable silence and stillness filled the room. I turned and looked at the picture of my father. He was luminous. A ray of light came from him and filled the entire room. It no longer seemed like a picture. It felt as if he was there.

Master Patanjali is saying that we will have moments in our lives that are full of light, and that light, in whatever way it comes to you, will remove the darkness in your life.

Going Forward in a Boat

तस्य वाचकः प्रणवः ॥ २७ ॥

tasya vācakaḥ praṇavaḥ

The sound of Isvara is AUM.
At the back of the whole creation is harmony.

—MASTER PATANJALI'S *YOGA SUTRAS*,
BOOK ONE, SUTRA 27

Master Patanjali describes AUM—that which is indescribable—by using the Sanskrit word *pranavah.* Like most words, *pranavah* has numerous meanings. *Pra* means to go forward and *nava* means boat. So AUM is to go forward in a boat. Going forward in a boat gives a sense of renewal. Renewal comes from praising others. Saying good things about others contains the sound of AUM.

Recently, David Life and Sharon Gannon were in New York teaching yoga classes for one week. I attended their classes with several hundred others. I found that since I'd been in the yoga community for so long, I knew many of the people in the class, and so found myself making a good many introductions.

While I was talking with Jeff, for instance, Giselle came up to me.

"Giselle," I said. "Do you know Jeff?"

"No," she replied.

"Jeff teaches yoga at Beth Israel hospital on the cancer and surgery floors," I continued. "He works with very sick people. He was trained at the Urban Zen Foundation, Donna Karan's organization, which works with teachers of yoga and meditation and teaches them how to be of service in hospitals. Jeff has told me that through restorative poses and simple movements the patients feel much better. He also says that through breath-awareness meditation, the patients become deeply relaxed. Everyone at the hospital speaks very highly of him. Several years ago, I was in Colombia with Jeff, where I was giving a workshop in Bogotá and he came as my student. At one point, I was teaching yoga to soldiers. Most of them were missing at least one limb. I was overwhelmed. Jeff stepped in for me; he wasn't overwhelmed at all. Giselle, please meet Jeff."

Giselle and Jeff immediately became friends. In this manner, I made many introductions during that week of teachings.

I found that when I was praising Jeff, it was no longer about me. It was all about Jeff. I had made myself small, and in doing that, I felt large. In his sermon known as the "Drum Major Instinct," given at Ebenezer Baptist Church in Atlanta Georgia on February 4, 1968, just two months before he was assassinated, Dr. Martin Luther King, Jr. requested that at his funeral the eulogizers not mention that he had "a Nobel Peace Prize—that isn't important. . . . I want you to be able to say that I did try to feed the hungry, to clothe those who were naked, to visit those who were in prison, to love and serve humanity."

On the acknowledgments page of my book *An Offering of Leaves,* I thanked my husband, whom I referred to as "a humble tai chi master." When he read that, he was upset. "Ruth, I'm not a master," he told me. "My teacher is a master." He wanted to see if I could have it removed from the text and asked me to call the publisher. I told him it was too late, and that the books were being printed as we spoke. He would have been happier had I described him as, "a dedicated student."

About the Author

Ruth Lauer Manenti is the daughter of Lothar and Stefanie Lauer. Her parents came to the United States from Europe as refugees. Her father was a scientist and her mother is a painter and a writer of short stories and novels. Ruth found her way to yoga twenty-five years ago after spending a year in bed due to a serious car accident. She has been teaching yoga for the past twenty years to students from around the world, primarily at the Jivamukti Yoga School in New York City. Ruth is a devoted student and has the blessings of her teachers: Sri K. Pattabhi Jois, Saraswathi Jois, Sharath Jois, Dr. M. A. Jayashree, Prof. M. A. Narasimhan, Prof. Nagaraja Rao, and Dr. Gurudat and his family. She is especially thankful to David Life and Sharon Gannon for being her teachers and also for giving her one of the most beautiful jobs in the world, the job of being a yoga teacher. Ruth's husband Robert is a nurse and they live in a cabin in the woods at the foot of the Catskill mountains. Ruth also has an MFA from the Yale School of Art.

Donation

In 2008, a non-profit organization was set up called Friends of Mysore Children, Inc. to help pay for doctors' bills, medicine, rice, clothes, computer courses, music lessons, books, and school supplies for people in need whom we met. Children still go every day to my friend Shakunthala's little store in Mysore. They sit on the floor while she feeds them and teaches them English. The children who mostly live in the streets have a place to go that is clean and safe where they are given love and affection.

I wish to thank everyone who has given to Friends of Mysore Children. All who gave did so because they wanted to, when no one was looking, outside of the spotlight. It has created a momentum of taking care of others, some so sad and so often ignored that they might otherwise have slipped through the cracks.

We changed our name from Friends of Mysore Children, Inc. to Saraswati's Hands. This was done to honor Saraswathi, Sri K. Pattabhi Jois' daughter, our Indian mother, and also to expand our description from a child in a city in India to really anyone. Everyone everywhere needs help at some time.

A portion of the proceeds from this book will go to Saraswati's Hands. If you would like to make an additional donation, please send to:

Saraswati's Hands
c/o Ruth Lauer Manenti
470 Stonybrook Road
Palenville, NY 12463

www.saraswatishands.org

Also by Ruth Lauer-Manenti

An Offering of Leaves
Lantern, 2009

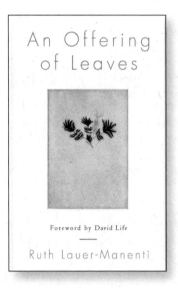